THE
UNWELCOME VISITOR

Also By Denise Welch

Starting Over
Pulling Myself Together
If They Could See Me Now
The Mother's Bond

Denise Welch is an actor and television personality. Among her TV credits are *Coronation Street* and *Waterloo Road*, alongside being a regular panellist on the ITV lunchtime chat show *Loose Women*. Denise has authored four previous books, both fiction and non-fiction.

THE
UNWELCOME VISITOR

Depression and How I Survive It

DENISE
WELCH

HODDER

First published in Great Britain in 2020 by Hodder & Stoughton
An Hachette UK company

This paperback edition published in 2021

1

. A CIP catalogue record for this title is available from the British Library

Paperback ISBN 9781529384574
eBook ISBN 9781529384581
Hardback ISBN 9781529384543

Typeset in Plantin Light by Hewer Text UK Ltd, Edinburgh
Printed and bound in Great Britain by Clays Ltd, Elcograf S.p.A.

Hodder & Stoughton policy is to use papers that are natural, renewable
and recyclable products and made from wood grown in sustainable
forests. The logging and manufacturing processes are expected to
conform to the environmental regulations of the country of origin.

Hodder & Stoughton Ltd
Carmelite House
50 Victoria Embankment
London EC4Y 0DZ

www.hodder.co.uk

For my mum, Annie.

The Unwelcome Visitor

Tonight I'm writing this message
As I feel myself going down
The usual signs are descending
My smiles are replaced by a frown

The world starts changing around me
And feels like a different place
I don't want to talk to my family
Don't want them to see my face

I'm tired and desperate for bedtime
But scared to go closing my eyes
The fear of tomorrow is on me
Don't want to see dark, dark skies

The visitor once more has come knocking
And uninvited lets himself in
I'll hide till he gets sick of waiting
As he knows I'll never give in

I don't know how long he'll be staying
But I'll sit it out just like before
It's painful, it hurts and I hate him
But I know he'll soon head for the door

I know I'm so loved and so cherished
And that is what gets me through
So if, like me, you're feeling frightened
Believe me, the sun will shine through

Denise Welch

Introduction

It is now more than thirty years since my visitor paid his first call, and he still comes to stay every now and then. I wish he wouldn't, because he's the very worst kind of guest. It makes no difference to him whether I'm happy or sad, weighed down by problems or fine; he turns up anyway, uninvited and unwelcome, and plunges me into a deep depression. I don't know why he's a 'he' or why he comes to suck away my joy and drain the colour from my life. All I know is that I hate having him around.

The unwelcome visitor doesn't come as frequently as he used to, thankfully. When he arrived in late September 2019, he hadn't been for six months, and I didn't give him a second thought as I got ready for a weekend road trip up to the north-east to stay with my sister, Debbie, and her three foster-children. I was driving up to Newcastle from Cheshire with my friend, Lisa, and her children, Pixie and Bella, and we were planning a weekend of fun. Debbie's foster-children and Pixie and Bella love seeing each other. It's always a fabulous, chaotic, crazy, screamy-screechy time when they get together.

I spent the Thursday before the trip in London, making one of my regular appearances on the TV talk show, *Loose Women*. In the evening, while I was on the train home to Cheshire, Lisa texted me to say that Pixie and Bella were beside themselves with excitement. 'Just to prepare you,' she wrote, 'they will want to play the 1975's music on full volume all the way up, especially "People", because the only time they're ever allowed to swear is when they sing it.'

Lisa was nanny to Louis, my youngest son, for many years, and a much-needed mother's help to me; my eldest son, Matthew, is godfather to one of her girls. She is quite a lot younger than me, but our lives have been entwined for fifteen years now.

'Can't wait!' I texted back, loving the idea of Pixie and Bella singing along with Matthew's band.

All was well with the world. I was really looking forward to the trip and there was nothing in me that was feeling unwell. If there had been, I would have had no problem ringing Lisa and saying, 'I'm too poorly to go,' because Lisa loves me and knows my illness very well. She would have gone ahead anyway, because she's very close to my sister, so there was no pressure on me to do the trip.

Friday came. We were going up in Lisa's car, and she and the girls came to get me. After waiting for the traffic to clear, off we went on our jolly way. Soon we were driving up the motorway, listening to Matthew's music. Some of the songs had shouty, sweary words and Lisa and I were in hysterics listening to the girls sing them.

We passed the Angel of the North and were nearing Newcastle when, in the midst of laughing with Lisa and the girls, the atmosphere in my head changed. Everything became less joyous. The colour started to bleed away from the world.

I wasn't thinking about anything in particular; I didn't say anything to make it happen. But life became greyer.

I carried on as normal. 'It'll go,' I thought. 'Just because I'm feeling like this doesn't mean the visitor is coming.'

Thoughts swirled in my head and I tried to reassure myself. 'Sometimes, if I get a good night's sleep, I'll wake up in the morning to find it's gone. Everything's going to be okay.'

We got to Debbie's house fairly late and I was hoping to have a cup of tea, make my excuses and go to bed. At the onset of illness, the main thing the depressive wants to do is withdraw from everything and everybody. That's why depression is the most isolating condition: you just want to be on your own.

I didn't say anything, because as soon as I say I'm not well, people become worried and upset for me. I didn't want to ruin anyone's evening; in any case, I was still hoping that I'd wake up in the morning and be fine.

The kids ran into the house and there was much joy and excitement at seeing their pals. Meanwhile, I walked into the kitchen to find Linda, one of my best north-eastern friends, sitting at the table. Normally, I would have been thrilled to sit down and chew the fat with Linda, Debbie and Lisa. I'd be having a cup of tea. They'd be having a glass of wine. We'd have a good catch-up.

Tonight, though, I didn't want to sit around chatting to the girls. I didn't want to talk to them at all. That told me I was heading for a fall.

Although I was desperate to go to bed, I stayed up and had a cup of tea. The others were talking about Greta Thunberg, and my sister said to me, 'I saw you liked something that Greta Thunberg posted – you, the woman who mixes up her recycling with her normal rubbish!'

Usually I would have said, 'What? Because I once threw a plastic carton out, now I can't support Greta Thunberg in her climate change campaign?' and this would have led to a bit of healthy banter between the two of us.

Instead, my sister's jokey comment felt like a barbed attack on me. Any kind of conflict makes me feel worse when I'm poorly. Other people I've spoken to who suffer from depression have said the same. In my mind, this was conflict. Yet it was just a comment.

I made my excuses and went to bed. 'Listen, girls, I'm knackered, and I've got a headache,' I said. 'I'm going to love you and leave you and go and lie down.'

Ordinarily, I love going to bed. It's where I watch far too much rubbish television, far too late at night, on my iPhone. It's a habit I'm trying to break, with little success, and so I nearly always fall asleep while one of my rubbish shows is still playing. It's just what I do! When I'm poorly, however, I have no desire whatever to watch back-to-back episodes of *90 Day Fiancé*, so instead I lay down in the dark and eventually drifted off to sleep.

When I awoke in the morning, the unwelcome visitor was there. I was engulfed in a thick, grey cloud of depression.

A couple of weeks earlier, I'd been at an inspirational awards dinner for people who had turned their lives around against the odds, and over dinner, I'd spoken to an Irish actress whose work I really admire. We'd had a lovely chat about everything under the sun, and when we said our goodbyes, she said, 'I'm so glad to have met you, Denise. I've had many issues with mental health and I follow everything you say and do. It's so important to me when you talk on social media about what you go through.'

'That's nice to hear, thank you!' I said.

It was an uplifting evening and I went to bed in a great mood. Later, when I looked at my phone, I could see that a few people had reached out to me on social media about being poorly. Since I was feeling well – and with the actress's words still in my head – I held my phone up and filmed myself saying something like, 'Hi guys, there seems to be something in the air tonight. People are struggling a bit and reaching out. You all know that I live with occasional visits from the unwelcome visitor . . . The most important thing to know is that he will leave.'

It was a 30-second video, but the next morning there were messages from people saying things like, 'I've watched this video ten times already. It has helped me so much!'

I was moved by the responses. 'It takes so little to make an impact,' I thought. 'I'm not giving anybody any clues as to how to get better. I'm just talking about my illness.'

Two weeks later, when I woke up in the middle of an episode at my sister's house, it was all I could do to have a shower in the morning. Just getting out of bed is hard with depression, as anyone who has experienced this illness will know. But I took a moment to think about the day ahead with Lisa, Debbie and the children, and I made myself get up. We were taking the kids to a trampoline park and having pizza for lunch; Debbie and I were also intending to have a catch-up about family matters. I didn't want to let anybody down.

I'm very good at knowing the level of my depression. This wasn't a crippling depression, but it was nonetheless the kind of grey depression that would make it extremely hard just to get through the day. Still, I was going to do it, for the sake of my family.

I had a shower and washed my hair. 'I want people who don't understand depression to know what this feels like,' I thought. 'You know what? I'm always posting about the joys and successes of my life. I'm going to show the other side of my life, right now.'

I picked up my phone and said, 'I want to share the bad times with you, so, here I am in the midst of a mild episode of clinical depression . . .'

I wasn't telling people about something that might happen. I wasn't on *Loose Women* talking about something that had happened. I was showing people how it feels, *now, this minute*, to have mild depression. (If it had been severe, I would not have been able to pick up the phone and video it.)

I tried to explain the sense of flatness and void that comes with an episode of depression. I posted another video fifteen minutes later, by which time I was in tears. 'Part of me feels ridiculous, sharing this . . .' I sobbed on the second video. 'But if I'm going to talk about the journey of an episode, I want you to see what's wrong with me. There's nothing different in my circumstances to yesterday, but now I'm terrified about everything, and everything is dark.'

I posted the video without thinking about the impact it would have. It didn't seem like a big deal to me. 'People ask me what it's like when the unwelcome visitor comes. Here's how it feels,' I thought.

A few hours later we were at the trampoline park, watching the kids having the time of their lives, and Debbie said, 'Are you okay?'

'I'm not, Debbie, but I'm all right. I'm just having my thing,' I replied.

Sometimes I don't want to name it, so I call it 'my thing'.

'I thought something was up,' Debbie said.

I turned to Lisa. 'I'm so sorry. I really was looking forward to this weekend, and I just feel I'm a complete downer.'

'For goodness' sake, don't be ridiculous!' Lisa said.

It's good to be reminded that it doesn't really affect other people when I'm feeling ill, because they're not the poorly ones. Yes, they feel sorry for me, but I've stopped having the weight of the world on me when it comes to how my illness affects other people. They had a great time at the trampoline park. The kids didn't know a thing.

Just before we left, I picked up my phone and saw a massive number of responses to my earlier posts. 'Oh no, what have I done? What are they saying?' I thought, panicking. I had never seen so many responses to anything I'd posted before.

I started to read through the comments. There were hundreds of responses from people who had depression, and their comments were touching, supportive and wonderful. Some were heartbreaking. There were other, equally moving comments that said things like, 'You have helped me understand my friend's depression,' or 'I've got a better idea of what my daughter goes through, thank you.'

There were also a few comments that said, 'I've never been very sympathetic to people with depression, really, but seeing it in real time has made me reconsider.'

Responses like these had a huge impact on me.

My husband, Lincoln, phoned to see how I was. He was concerned that I had put myself in a situation that would make me worse, because I take on the worries of the world. He's often concerned about that.

'No, I don't regret it,' I told him.

Lisa, the kids and I drove back down to Cheshire the next day. 'I'm not going to be great company, so pop your music on,' I said.

Having known Lisa for so long, I didn't need to put on a false front. I slept for a lot of the journey. When I wasn't asleep, I sat with my eyes closed to create the sense that I was alone. Lisa was fine and the girls were playing in the back. Life was going on.

I got home to an empty house and was glad to be on my own. I looked at my phone and experienced a sudden wave of sorrow for everybody who has depression, including myself. I felt desperately sad that I've had this illness for so many years.

Conscious that I'd said I would go on posting through the episode, I filmed myself crying. But after I posted it, I thought, 'Oh God, have I done the right thing? Am I going to lose work over this?'

'You know, I don't care,' I decided. 'I promised to be honest to people, so I will be.'

After the response I'd had to my first two posts, sharing my experience of depression had become more important to me than any job. It didn't matter to me if some people thought I was weak, or a nutter, or if they were thinking, 'What on earth is she doing? Why would we want to see her crying face?'

I wanted to share the other side of my life, because you can see a lot of fake 'perfect' lives on social media, and many social media users live in a compare-and-despair world, unhappy that their lives don't match up to other people's fictitious lives. It's wonderful to share highlights of your life on the different platforms – I do it – but it's terrible that people believe others have a perfect life, when they don't. So it's important to say, 'A lot of the time I have a great life, and I share it with you. But I also have to cope with this side of my life.'

The depression started to lift the next day, but the team at *Loose Women* were obviously concerned about me and I took a few days off work. My producer, Sally, rang me to tell me how proud she was that *Loose Women* had somebody speaking out on behalf of people who suffer this illness.

I've been talking publicly about depression for almost three decades now; I want to tell people with this illness that they are not alone, and explain how it feels to people who don't understand it. Those of us who have this illness are very good at masking the signs, but the signs are there. Showing people what depression looks like makes it much easier for them to identify it in their loved ones.

I thought long and hard about writing a book about my illness, because I knew that I would be revisiting very dark periods of my life that maybe I didn't want to think about again. But the importance of writing a book became paramount after my first post hit a million views. Mostly, I'm hoping this book will be a comfort to others who live with this illness, as I do. I think of us as a tribe, and we're a lot stronger than people might think. But I'm also aiming to help people who don't know about depression to understand it more.

People who would otherwise have said, 'What have you got to be depressed about? I don't get it!'

This is why you are reading *The Unwelcome Visitor* today.

PART 1

Post-natal Depression

I had never had a single day of any kind of psychiatric illness before my first child, Matthew, was born in 1989, when I was thirty-one. Years later, a psychologist insisted that he could have spotted signs that I was vulnerable to post-natal depression while I was pregnant, but I really doubt it. There were no signs.

When I became pregnant with Matthew, I was in a very happy relationship with a man I loved: the actor Tim Healy. Although Tim and I had only been together for six months and the pregnancy wasn't planned, we hadn't done much to prevent it and were overjoyed by the news that we were having a baby. We had some money in the bank, life was good and we both wanted a child. In the months leading up to Matthew's birth, we got married and began the process of buying a beautiful house in the north-east of England, where we had both grown up.

I had a fabulous pregnancy. I was the typical blooming pregnant woman that you read about: my skin was glowing, my hair was great and my eyes shining. The hormonal changes that were happening in my body made me feel fantastic and I was the envy of several other expectant women. I loved every minute of being pregnant and couldn't wait for the birth of our much-wanted child.

Tim and I were originally having an NHS birth at an old Victorian hospital in north London, a grim, dark, Gothic place where they kept losing my notes and I never saw the same person twice when I went for antenatal care. As the weeks passed, I felt less and less comfortable there: after they tried to treat me four times for the same minor ailment and repeatedly rang me to say, 'You've got an infection! Come in immediately!' I decided I wanted to go elsewhere to have our baby if at all possible.

So, although it was against our politics at the time, we changed to a private hospital, where I immediately felt a lot safer. Even when I went nine days overdue, there was no panic at all. My mum wasn't happy about it, but my obstetrician seemed very relaxed and I wasn't one of these mothers who was desperate for the baby to come out. I was still enjoying the whole process.

'There's another girl who's two weeks over and they're not doing anything,' I told my mum.

'Well, maybe they should be,' she said, gently.

The private hospital had been recommended by a friend who'd been treated for a non-pregnancy-related issue, so it was a while before I realised it was a natural birth centre. 'But pain relief will be available, won't it?' I asked at one of the prenatal classes I attended in the lead-up to the birth.

'Of course it will be, Mrs Healy!' I was assured. 'We're not living in Victorian times.'

Fast-forward to the labour, two months later, and nobody would give me any pain relief. 'Could somebody please do something to put me out of this agony?' I screamed. 'Hit me over the head with a spiked mallet! Anything!'

'But you're doing so well,' the midwives kept saying. 'You're nearly at the second stage of labour.'

The first stage of labour, known as 'established labour', usually lasts ten to twelve hours. Mine lasted forty-two hours. This is the period when you have regular, painful contractions while the cervix dilates from 3 centimetres to full dilation at 10 centimetres. My mum later told me that she thought it was inhumane of them not to give me anything to ease the pain – and she didn't like the idea of me being in labour for forty-two hours with an already overdue child, either. It was a very, very long forty-two hours.

There wasn't even gas and air available. Instead there was a load of trendy malarkey and the only pain relief I was offered was the chance to sit in a birthing pool, which was just a blow-up bath, really, a kids' paddling pool.

The warm water seemed to help a little, at first. Then Tim said, 'Do you mind if I go out for a fag?'

Unfortunately, just after he left the birthing-pool room, a lightbulb exploded and I suddenly found myself alone in total darkness. My contractions were agonising, I was vomiting into the water; I panicked. 'Help!' I shouted. 'Someone, please come and get me out of here!'

It was a comedy of errors, but I didn't find much to laugh about at the time. The only good bit I can remember is the final hour of that first stage of labour, which I spent back in my private room leaning over a trendy beanbag watching the *Dynasty* spin-off, *The Colbys*, on the television. It was around the time when *Dynasty* started to become completely ridiculous and in this episode Fallon was being captured by aliens. Despite the pain and discomfort I was in, I was so enthralled by the turn of events that when the midwife came in to break my waters, I said, 'Wait! Just give me a couple of minutes to see what happens . . .'

As the credits rolled, she broke my waters and triggered the second stage of labour, which is supposed to take an hour. Mine lasted seven hours.

I had no bearing-down reflex and wasn't getting the pushing right. 'Are you sure you haven't still got your tights on?' Tim asked, attempting to inject some humour into a difficult situation.

I can laugh about it now, but jokes like that don't always go down very well at the time.

A lot of people have since said to me that the hospital should never have let the second stage of my labour go to seven hours, not least because of the danger it posed to my baby. They weren't clamouring to get him out after seven hours, either, so goodness knows how long they would have let it go on for. Eventually, I was able to push, thank God, and gave birth to Matthew in the squat position – again, so trendy! He was born on the floor, a healthy eight-pound baby boy, and suddenly everything was wonderful.

'I suppose a fuck's out of the question?' quipped Tim, ever the joker.

Having just pushed out a baby, you can imagine the look I gave him!

I was delighted to have a boy. Many women seem to want to have a girl the first time round, but my vision of my child was of a little boy. One of the happiest moments of my life was phoning my parents to tell them Matthew had arrived. It was something I had always looked forward to doing.

There were only five or six women having babies in the hospital, so there were plenty of nurses around to help. It felt a bit like a hotel, really. Each room had an emergency cord, but I never needed mine. 'You're the only one who hasn't pulled the cord,' the nurses told me. 'You're such a natural mother.'

The breastfeeding side of things wasn't working too well, though: Matthew was very hungry and crying a lot. But I wasn't anxious, assuming we'd both get the hang of it.

I had Matthew on the Saturday and they said I could go home on the Wednesday, so I had a few blissful days of holding him and bonding with him before we left. We had some friends in, but I didn't want loads of people visiting: I wanted all of that to happen when we got home. I was really excited that Mum and Dad were coming to stay later on in the week and couldn't wait to introduce them to their first grandchild.

On the Wednesday, Tim and I got Matthew ready, put him in his little carrycot and off we went. I felt fine as we drove through north London, an area I knew well because I had lived there for ten years, and yet the drive felt like something out of a dream, as if I was on the outside looking in. I didn't question it because I thought it was probably normal for things to feel a little surreal just after having a baby. It is a huge life change. You arrive at hospital with no baby and you leave with a baby, thinking, 'I can't believe this baby is mine!'

We arrived home at our flat in Highgate, where there was a mountain of cards and flowers waiting. I felt very emotional reading all the lovely messages people had written. I couldn't help crying when I read words like, 'Welcome home, Mum!'

It was overwhelming, but in a nice way. 'Oh God, I can't stop crying,' I sobbed.

'You've got the baby blues,' Tim kept saying.

There was nothing untoward about it: as many as 80 per cent of women get the baby blues during the fortnight after giving birth, when they feel a bit sad and emotional as their levels of pregnancy hormones rapidly drop. I had a bit of a restless night later, because Matthew didn't sleep too well, but that was also to be expected and I wasn't worried. I still wasn't doing very well with the breastfeeding and didn't feel that he was getting what he needed from my boobs, but I was learning, and I was okay.

I woke up on the Thursday morning, after not much sleep. Mum and Dad were arriving in the afternoon, and my mum and dad seeing my firstborn child was a moment that I'd dreamt about since I was sixteen. I'd always had this romantic notion of my parents seeing their grandchild for the first time.

When they arrived, Mum took one look at Matthew and was overwhelmed by love. It completely blindsided her and she started crying. 'I always knew that I would love my grandchild, because he's your child, but I am completely and utterly blown away by the force of emotion that I feel for him,' she told me, adding that it was almost akin to her love for my sister, Debbie, and me.

I didn't feel the way I'd thought I was going to feel at this longed-for moment. I was aware of some disconnect, a deadening of my emotions. 'I feel a bit weird,' I thought, but tried not to show it. I had a strong desire to be on my own, which was very unlike me, so I yawned and said I felt tired and went off to bed quite early, after having something to eat.

A few hours later, I woke up with a start to find myself in the middle of an intense, terrifying panic attack. I was gasping for breath and my heart was racing to the point that it felt cartoon-like, something out of *Tom and Jerry*, when their hearts jump out of their chests. I had no idea what was happening. I had never experienced anything like it before.

It was the kind of panic and anxiety you feel if you're driving along on the motorway and a car suddenly pulls out in front of you. You think you're going to crash: your heart rate speeds up and keeps on racing even after the situation resolves itself and you don't crash.

You pull over to the hard shoulder, punch the steering wheel and shout, 'Fucking hell!'

You give yourself five minutes, you calm down, your heartbeat slows and you're on your way again.

That's how I felt when I woke up gasping for breath, except that my heart didn't ever really slow down, and every time Matthew made even the smallest mew it would start racing again. I was up most of the night after that. I probably only got another hour's sleep.

When I came to in the morning, my whole lactation process had stopped. My boobs were flat like a spaniel's ears; my milk had gone and I couldn't feed my baby. Six days after having Matthew, I had nothing to give him.

I now know that this was a major sign of massive hormone imbalance, but I had no point of reference at the time. Nobody had warned me that it might happen and I had next to no knowledge of post-natal illness. It just felt as if I was losing the plot.

Thank God for my mum. 'Let's talk to the midwife when she comes,' she soothed. 'I'm sure this is completely normal. It's only your second night at home.'

Mum was amazing and I was so lucky to have her there, because not only was she my wonderful, loving mother, but she was also a trained psychiatric nurse, so she knew exactly what to say. Even though she was secretly worried, she made all the right noises to calm me down.

There was no continuity of care from the private hospital where I'd had Matthew and so it was a community midwife who visited later that day.

'I feel terrible,' I told her. 'I don't feel anxious about the fact that I have a baby, but my body is having a panic attack and my lactation has stopped.'

'Oh, that's very unusual,' the midwife said with a frown, the very words you *don't* want to hear when you're a new mother. 'That normally only happens if a spouse or a parent dies.'

I looked at her helplessly. Instead of bringing comfort and support, she seemed very detached and businesslike, almost uncaring.

'Anyway, there's nothing you can do about it,' she went on briskly. 'You'll just have to go out and get some bottles and feed baby with a bottle.'

'That's it?' I asked.

I'm sure she had a million babies and mothers to see that day, but I had expected more of a midwife.

'Well, yes! There's nothing we can do. You haven't got any milk. Good luck,' she said, and she was gone.

While Tim went out and got the bottles, milk and steriliser, Mum said lots of lovely, encouraging things to help me feel better about not breastfeeding. 'I'm all for bottle-feeding,' she said. 'Bottle-fed babies sleep better, and the formula is so amazing these days, and having bottles means we can all join in and help you.'

I tried to smile. Tim came back with the bottles and soon Matthew was feeding hungrily. 'I'm not going to get obsessed with the fact that I can't breastfeed,' I kept telling myself.

I must have seemed okay the following day, because Dad and Tim went off to play golf. In the afternoon, Mum said, 'Should we take him out for a walk?'

I remember thinking, 'I don't really want to go for a walk, but I will, because it's what I'm supposed to do.'

It was the first time I'd taken Matthew out and we put him in his pram and walked down to Crouch End, an area that I'd known for years because it's where I went to drama school. Again, I had that feeling of unreality. 'It's like I'm in a dream,' I told Mum.

'Oh, that's completely normal,' she said.

We went to a cafe and sat down for a cup of tea. 'I feel weird, Mum,' I said, 'I want my reality to come back. I've lived here for ten years and yet it feels like I'm not connecting to the world.'

'You don't feel depressed, do you?' she asked, ever alert to signs of mental illness.

'No, I don't feel depressed, just disconnected.'

This was the moment that Mum really started to worry, she later told me.

On the way back home, we stopped at a newsagent's to get some milk: Mum stayed outside while I went in to buy it. It was 15 April 1989 and the first reports of the Hillsborough disaster were coming through on the radio.

When I came out of the shop, I said, 'My God, Mum. This terrible thing's happened in Hillsborough and ninety-six people have been killed. It's just awful.'

Mum was horrified and we walked the half a mile back to the flat in near silence. 'Did they say how it happened?' she asked as we were arriving home.

'Oh Mum, that was just a dream,' I said dismissively. 'I told you I had a dream about it.'

'You didn't, pet,' Mum replied. 'You told me about it when you came out of the shop just now.'

'No, it was a dream!' I insisted. 'Stop trying to make me think I'm going mad.'

At that, Mum knew something was seriously wrong.

Half an hour later my two great friends, Lester and Paul, arrived to see the baby. Lester was being his customary hilarious self, taking the mickey out of me and asking whether I'd be going out dancing that night?

This had been a running joke among my friends while I was pregnant, because I was known as the go-to person for fun and frivolity. 'Oh yes, she'll be out at a nightclub four days after the birth!' Lester used to say, and we'd all laugh. 'The baby will be handed to the guy who delivers the Yellow Pages and she'll be out to a disco.'

Now Lester and Paul were trying their best to make me laugh again, but I couldn't even smile. These were people I was normally desperate to see, but now I was desperate for them to leave.

'I want them to go,' I thought, and as the words swirled around my head, a terrible blackness crept up my body and I was filled with the darkest despair. Within thirty seconds, I was engulfed by a suicidal, pitch-black mental depression.

I only have a vague memory of what happened next because I was slipping in and out of lucidity. I know that Mum saw Lester and Paul to the door and when she came back in she found me at the window, climbing on a chair to get onto the windowsill. I'm not sure what I was trying to do, but Mum thought I was trying to jump out and pulled me back from the window. She immediately called the hospital where I'd had the baby and, when Tim and Dad came home from playing golf, they found two hospital medics at my bedside, at a loss as to how to help me.

The unwelcome visitor had arrived to pay his first call and my life had changed for ever.

II

Post-natal depression is the cruellest, most unforgiving and isolating condition, because not only are you submerged in a pitch-black nightmare of mental illness, but you also have a totally dependent child who can't survive without you. You don't want to do anything – you've hardly got the energy or the will to get through the day – yet you have this helpless baby to look after.

It is such a confusing time, because you are no longer the person you were. Depression robs you of everything you know and everything you feel. I can see it in people's faces sometimes, when they're staring into the distance and there's nothing in their eyes, just a void. The best way I can describe it is like having a vice in your head. You are completely numb and cut off from the world; you can't feel anything.

After depression overwhelmed me, I became a woman in a dressing gown, unable to cope with responsibility for anything. I was lucky to have the support of my family, because everything was so dark and bewildering that I couldn't have functioned on my own with a child. It is horrible to imagine a single parent alone in a tenement block with a new baby, feeling as I did. How on earth would they manage? My heart goes out to anyone suffering from severe post-natal depression who doesn't get the help or understanding they need.

Thankfully, my mum forced me to feed Matthew myself, knowing how important it was to keep our physical contact going. Those early days of a child's life are crucial and Matthew and I needed to share the smell, touch, warmth and familiarity that bond a mother and her baby. I'm so grateful that Mum had the knowledge, foresight and love to make me do it. It meant that Matthew didn't suffer, because he had me feeding him and holding him, and when I looked back on those early weeks with him, I didn't think, 'But I never even fed him!'

Every four hours, Mum would say to me, 'It's time to go and get the bottles.'

Oh, but it was a lot easier said than done. Our attic flat in Highgate had an open-plan kitchen/living area and the whole room was about thirty feet long. I can remember sitting on the sofa at one end of the room and seeing the Milton bottles and the steriliser in the far distance at the other end: they seemed so far away and so impossible to reach that it was the equivalent of someone saying, 'There's Kilimanjaro. Go and climb it.'

'Can you . . . ?' I'd say to Mum.

'No, I want you to do it,' she'd reply.

So I would heave myself off the sofa and walk like an automaton along to the kitchen, where I'd carefully make up a bottle with powder and sterilised water. Then I'd walk robotically back again, sit down and hold Matthew and feed him, feeling absolutely nothing. Not love, not hate, just nothing.

It doesn't sound possible, does it – to feel nothing whatsoever? But that's what depression is – it depresses your emotions so that you can't feel anything, good or bad. When I'm depressed, it would make no difference to me if someone knocked on my door to say that I had just won a hundred million pounds on the Lottery, or if they came to tell me that my entire family had been wiped out in an aeroplane crash. I would feel nothing, either way. It is hard to imagine if you've never experienced it, but that's how it is.

The drop in my hormones had probably affected my lactation early on and I suspect that my breasts had never been feeding Matthew properly, but as soon as he started being bottle fed, he was a really great baby, thankfully. He didn't cry very much and slept brilliantly, so he wasn't a cause for worry.

I slept a lot, too: I longed for oblivion because my days were a living hell and the only time I felt normal was when I was asleep. I was living in a reverse nightmare: instead of waking up from a bad dream and thinking, 'Thank God!', I'd have normal dreams during the night and open my eyes in the morning, thinking, 'Oh no, I'm back in the nightmare.'

I desperately wanted somebody to give me an injection to make the pain go away. 'Could I go to hospital to be put out?' I asked Mum.

You know when you have a general anaesthetic and they tell you to count down? 'Ten, nine, eight, seven . . .' and then you're out? That's all I wished for.

Tim had two acting jobs at the time and was under a lot of pressure: he had to leave on the Sunday to start rehearsals for a series called *Boon* with Michael Elphick in Birmingham, and then get in a car to drive through the night to Bristol to film *Casualty*. His acting commitments meant that he wasn't going to be at home very much for several weeks, which would have been fine if I'd been well, but was catastrophic now. I couldn't be left alone, so my mum decided to stay and look after me. She rang her boss and put in for six weeks' unpaid leave from work, bless her.

In the days and weeks that followed, Mum spent hours sitting by my bed, stroking my hand and giving me constant reassurance. Engulfed by depression, I was like a child again. 'But you do love me more than you love Matthew, don't you?' I'd say.

It seems incomprehensible to me now that I would be thinking in such a way. I was thirty-one years old, not ten!

'Of course, darling,' Mum said, again and again. 'I could never love anybody more than I love you and your sister.'

'Why am I having these ridiculous feelings about my mum loving my son more than me, when he's just a baby?' I thought anxiously. 'Who does that?'

There is a smell I associate very strongly with that time: Mum's perfume, Ivoire by Balmain, which was the only perfume she had brought with her to London for the couple of days she had originally been planning to stay. It has a gorgeous scent, but there was a long period when it could set my heart racing if I happened to walk past someone who was wearing it, because it was so reminiscent of that time when I didn't know who I was.

The hospital where I'd had Matthew wanted me to go in for an assessment, but Mum thought it would be better for me to see my GP first. Since I wasn't capable of ringing up and making an appointment, she arranged for me to go on the Monday morning. It was a monumental effort for me to wash and get dressed to go out. After I'd showered, I sat on a corner of the sofa in my dressing gown, staring zombie-like into space, while Mum handed me my clothes.

When I was finally ready, we went the short distance to the doctor's in a taxi. I felt very poorly and scared on the journey; I felt so bad that, as we were pulling away from a set of traffic lights, I opened the car door and would have thrown myself out if Mum hadn't grabbed me and pulled me back. I don't know what I was thinking at that moment. I'm sure I wasn't trying to kill myself, but anybody who has been depressed will know that you'll do anything to stop the pain in your head. You're not thinking rationally about wanting to die. Most people who take their own lives don't actually want to die; they just want to stop the pain.

The GP surgery where I was registered was one of those big practices with lots of doctors, where you never see the same doctor twice. The GP we saw was probably around the age I am now, but to me at the time she looked at least ninety-seven.

My mum did most of the talking for me, because I was practically catatonic and could barely say anything.

'I want to hear *you* talking,' the doctor kept saying.

'It's depression. I'm so depressed,' I said eventually.

Without a flicker of sympathy, she leant forward, looked me squarely in the eye and said, 'Well, I had five children, dear, and I just didn't have time to get depressed.'

I still can't quite believe she said those words, even though I have been quoting them for the last thirty years and they are burned on my psyche and emblazoned on my soul. Where was the sympathy, the understanding? I was a first-time mum who had no history of mental illness and had been perfectly fine until only a few days before, but was now so poorly that I could hardly speak.

I knew exactly what Mum was thinking. 'Don't you dare say that you had five children and didn't have time to get depressed! This is a very sick girl who just tried to throw herself out of a taxi.'

Mum was furious. 'If I ever see her in the street, God help her,' she fumed as we left the surgery.

The doctor prescribed antidepressants, which helped a little, at least. They must have had a sedative effect because, in my longing for sleep, I counted down the minutes to each dose. I was always asking Mum, 'When can I have my tablets?'

'In just a little while,' she'd say. 'Not long to go.'

After our disastrous visit to the GP, Mum phoned the hospital where I'd had Matthew and arranged for me to see the doctor who delivered him. This doctor was well known and very popular with celebrities and royals (as I discovered later), so he was clearly a master tradesman. But when I went to see him, expecting him to confirm that I had post-natal depression and talk about possible ways of treating it, he decided to play amateur psychologist with me, which he wasn't qualified to do, in my opinion.

He took me into a room in the hospital maternity unit, next to where I'd had the baby, laid me down on a bed and put a cover over my eyes. Then, to my consternation, he started talking about the two abortions I'd had when I was younger.

'You have to forgive yourself,' he intoned. 'You must put these things in the past and move on.'

It was the last thing I'd expected him to say – and it created the most massive anxiety in me. Not in a month of Sundays had it occurred to me that the way I was feeling could be connected to having an abortion, but that's what he was trying to pin it to. Like the GP before him, he was basically saying that it was my own fault that I was ill, perhaps to shift my focus away from the failings of the hospital: 'It's nothing to do with us – it's you.'

It left me thinking, 'Is it me? Am I to blame?'

Considering that women have been giving birth since the beginning of human history, it still amazes me to think that so little was known about post-natal depression until so recently. This was a doctor who had delivered hundreds of babies and must have come across post-natal illness many times in his patients, and yet he didn't seem to have a clue about what had caused it or how to go about treating it. (In a horrible footnote to what I went through at the natural birth hospital where I had Matthew, the other overdue mum on my ward that I'd told my mum about was allowed to go four weeks past her due date and gave birth to a stillborn baby.)

Mum was appalled when she heard what the obstetrician had been saying to me and even less impressed when he sent us off to see a cranial osteopath. Never having heard of cranial osteopathy, I went along assuming I'd be seeing a brain specialist, only to have my neck twisted around by a man who claimed to be balancing the rhythmic pulses flowing through my head. It was desperate. I had something in my physical system that was so black and oppressive that I couldn't function. Anybody who thought that it could be cured by massaging my neck had to be off their rocker.

'No one understands,' I told Mum despairingly. 'I'm never going to get better.'

'Yes, you will,' she said steadfastly. 'You will get better.'

I think the idea of suicide would have been in my mind at that moment if not for Mum, because the feeling that nobody understands what you're going through is so painful and isolating.

Mum never once said to me, 'What do you think's brought this on?' In her mind, I'd had a baby and it had made me very poorly. That was all there was to it. Her focus was, 'What can we do to get her better?'

But it was beginning to feel as if I had nowhere to turn to find a cure for my illness. All the doctors I saw around this time assumed that I had a psychological problem that stemmed from self-indulgence or guilt – or even suspected childhood trauma. It was unsettling how quickly they jumped to their conclusions. None of them would agree that the problem was physical. They insisted that they knew better than we did because of their medical qualifications.

I felt abandoned. I needed information and medical support, but it was nowhere to be found. I scoured every parent and baby magazine I could get my hands on, but they just showed new mums having an amazing, happy time, gazing adoringly at their babies and laughing in parks.

Eventually, I came across a magazine containing a list of ailments that might afflict a mum and her baby after the birth. It was an exhaustive list, detailing *every possible* condition the writers could think up in their wildest imaginings, almost to the point where they were saying, 'If your child is born with ten ears, ring this number.' 'If you develop another nose, call this number for help and advice.'

I scanned the pages in desperation. There was no mention of post-natal depression.

Then, at last, right down at the bottom of the page, in a tiny box in the left-hand corner, I saw the words: 'If you think that you have something more than the baby blues, contact the Association for Post-Natal Illness at this address.'

There was no phone number. You had to write to them. That was all the help there was. I still wonder how many letters they received, because writing a letter when you're severely depressed feels like an impossible task. With my mum's assistance, I wrote away and I think they may have sent a leaflet back. It was a relief to know that I wasn't the only person in the country suffering from depression after having a baby, but it wasn't enough. As well as knowing that I wasn't alone, I needed reassurance that I was going to get better. I needed to know that one day this thick, black cloud would disappear.

These days, when I have a depressive episode I comfort myself with the thought that it will pass, however grim, vile or frightening it is at the time. But I didn't know anything about psychiatric illness then: I used the word 'depressed' in the way that most people do, because they don't know what it's like to have real depression. I used to say I was 'depressed' by the weather when it was grey and rainy; I used to say I was 'depressed' if I didn't get a job I wanted. When circumstances dictated, I felt low and down, but I had never experienced severe anxiety or clinical depression.

I would have given anything to see a woman come on the television and talk about having my illness. Someone who was well, who had a couple of children and could smile and say, 'I had what you had. I've been where you are right now. But look at me now. Yes, I still have it, but in between I live this great life with my two children. You will get better.'

But back then people didn't feel like they could talk about it, so no one did.

I don't know what I would have done without my mum's reassurance. 'You will get better,' she told me, every single day, even though she can't have known the full truth of that.

I needed to hear those words more than anything, and so they are the words I always say to people who tell me they have depression: 'You will get better.'

It has become my mantra. 'You will get better.'

I was very fortunate that none of my close family ever questioned that I had a severe mental illness. They knew I wasn't the type of person to indulge in a condition that wasn't there. They never saw it as an indulgence or a neurosis, as some others did, and yet it must have been very hard to understand, because it appeared out of nowhere and took over so quickly and absolutely.

It was an awful time for Tim. He was desperately worried about me and hated being away. He phoned as often as he could, but instead of hearing joyful news of baby's progress, all he got was me sobbing hysterically and talking about wanting to take my own life. When he came home after ten days away, he was alarmed to see how pale and thin I looked. My appetite had vanished and I was finding it hard to swallow. I'd lost a stone and a half and seemed to be wasting away.

Poor Tim. His fun-loving, happy-go-lucky wife had been replaced by a lifeless figure on the sofa, staring into space. I just wasn't the person he had married.

I constantly complained of a sense of unreality. 'This doesn't feel like our flat,' I told him. 'Nothing feels the same.'

It didn't help that he walked in sporting a moustache, which he'd grown for his part playing a seedy nightclub comic in *Boon*. It made me feel anxious to look at him. 'Why is everything changing? Why do you have to look different?' I kept asking him.

I was aware of the reality of the situation, but any tiny change made things feel even more surreal than they already were. It got so bad that he had to talk to me with his hand over his mouth to hide the moustache. Then, whenever he took his hand away, I'd say, 'Why do you keep changing?'

I now know that I was on the verge of a puerperal psychosis, a horrendous post-natal illness that can trigger mania, delusions, hallucinations and paranoia in the weeks after giving birth. Women who have puerperal psychosis in its fully fledged form don't know who they are or who the baby is; they have suicidal urges and some of them have feelings that they want to hurt their baby. It's a psychiatric emergency.

Things never got that bad for me, but I was close. I can recall everything, so I was lucid, and I never wanted to harm Matthew – but I can also remember looking down at him in his carrycot next to me and thinking, 'Why is that baby here?'

It gives me the shivers when I read the tragic headlines about mothers who kill themselves, partly because I came within a millimetre of losing all sense of reality after I had Matthew, but also because there's so little understanding of this horrendous illness. It really upsets me when I come across people who are judgemental about the awful cases that are reported in the news. 'Did you read about that woman who walked into the sea off the beach at Brighton?' they'll say. 'Look at that – how selfish! She had everything – a loving husband, two gorgeous babies, a beautiful home and her own business – how could she have done such a thing?'

My first thought when I read a tragic story on these lines will always be that perhaps the woman in question had post-natal illness. Often she is described as the perfect wife and daughter, and a loving mother. She has never been known to say a bad word about anybody, but then she suddenly turns into a 'devil woman'. It is horrific. People can have no idea what it took for her to take her own life.

Fortunately, puerperal psychosis is rare. If post-natal

depression affects at least one in ten women (and probably a lot more, because many cases go unreported or undiagnosed) then the one in a thousand women suffering from puerperal psychosis doesn't sound like very many. Then again, with around 2,000 births a day in the UK, it suddenly adds up to more than ten new cases a week, which isn't insignificant.

I get a better picture of it when I think of it visually. At a mums' and babies' show at a theatre the size of the Palace Theatre, Manchester, say, or the Hippodrome, Birmingham, there would be two women suffering from puerperal psychosis in the audience, at least 200 suffering from varying degrees of post-natal depression and anything up to 1,600 with the baby blues! Motherhood, eh? Imagine how different things would be if men gave birth: there would have to be a post-natal illness clinic on every corner, otherwise the world would grind to a halt.

The good news for women who suffer puerperal psychosis is that they can be very effectively treated with antidepressants, antipsychotic drugs and electric shock treatment. They usually go on to make a complete recovery within six weeks and never experience anything relating to it again, which is great. Not so post-natal depression, sadly – which is why, I have to admit, I used to half-wish I'd had puerperal psychosis.

Desperate to find help for me and underwhelmed by the doctors London had to offer, Mum decided that the best thing would be to take me home, where I could see a doctor who knew my family. I think she felt I would be far better off among no-nonsense northerners. So, with Tim's blessing, I took Matthew to stay at Mum and Dad's house in the village of Ebchester, near Consett, County Durham, where I had lived happily with my family between the ages of twelve and eighteen before setting off for drama school.

Tim was fine about me going home. He was just grateful that my parents could be there for me, because he was tired out from working all hours and worrying himself sick about me. He tells a story about how he had to act as though he'd had a heart attack as part of his job in *Casualty*. They took him into make-up, dusted his nose and said, 'Right, that's you.'

'What do you mean?' he said. 'I'm here to be made up for the next scene.'

The make-up artist took another look at him. 'Yup, all done,' she said. He looked so drained and ill that he didn't need any cosmetic help to look like a heart-attack patient!

It was a relief for Tim to know I was safe at home and I was glad to leave London. I felt calmer at home with Mum and Dad, although I was still living in a black void. I find it hard to recall those darkest of days because they were just so awful. More than anything, I wanted my feelings back: just to be able to experience emotions again, especially for my baby; just to be normal.

Even though I'm not religious in the least, I used to pray, 'To anything, to the universe, please, please, help me to love my baby.'

Years later, long after Matthew had grown up, he wrote the song 'She Lays Down' about these moments. It's on the album *I Like It When You Sleep, for You Are So Beautiful Yet So Unaware of It*, by his band, the 1975.

It's tough for me to listen to the song, because it's so heart-felt – and some of the lines are heartbreaking. 'She's appalled by not loving me at all,' he sings. 'She wears a frown and a dressing gown/When she lays down.'

The lyrics express exactly how I felt. I can remember lying on the floor with Matthew, looking at him and thinking, 'I just want to love this child.'

III

Someone recommended I see a psychiatrist. I think he might have been in London, possibly even in Harley Street, although I was so poorly at the time that I can't be sure. I just know that Tim would have paid any amount of money for me to go anywhere, to see anybody, if it would have made me better.

The psychiatrist had a very condescending sneer. 'Let's talk about your childhood,' he said.

'I had a very happy childhood,' I told him.

'Did you?' he asked, as if he didn't really believe me.

'This isn't to do with my childhood,' I said. 'I've had a baby. Something physical has changed in me. I think maybe my hormones have made me ill.'

That sneer again. 'Well, I can assure you that, in 99 per cent of cases, the cause of depression is rooted in childhood,' he said. 'Let's go back to some early memories. Do you remember anything particularly that might have upset you? Did your father spend too much time in the bathroom with you when you were young, for instance?'

He was laughably wide of the mark, but the way he was leading the conversation was very scary. It made me realise how easily people can be lured into having fake memories implanted in their minds when they are feeling vulnerable; JI can absolutely understand False Memory Syndrome. I escaped it, but I could feel that I was prone to it. I was so poorly and so desperate to get well that it was easy to imagine letting the seed be planted if I thought it would eventually lead, through psychiatric treatment, to release from depression.

I watch a lot of true-life crime programmes that focus on false confessions. With the right technique, it appears to be quite possible to persuade someone that they are guilty of a crime they haven't committed. Similarly, this psychiatrist wanted me to believe that my illness was something it wasn't, and that I was in denial about my past. His superior expression said, 'It will be something in your childhood. You'll realise it eventually.'

He wrote his phone number on a piece of paper and gave it to me. 'When you're ready to talk, come back again,' he said.

I have been cautious about psychiatrists ever since, even though I know there are some really good ones out there. Maybe I've just been unlucky, but too many mental health professionals have tried to press a troubled childhood onto me, when in fact I had a fantastic childhood and a very loving relationship with my parents.

Whenever I drive past our old family house in Monkseaton, Whitley Bay, it brings back incredibly happy memories of living there, and I loved living at our house in Ebchester, too. My parents had their ups and downs, but who doesn't? I'm sure we as a family had many of the problems that most families experience; I'm sure we were dysfunctional in many ways. Even so, I remember my years growing up as bathed in sunshine, love, friendship and community. I just can't imagine digging deep enough to find a psychological reason for my illness. I'd get to Australia first, I think.

When I went back to drama school in London for my second year, aged nineteen, and we talked about what we had got up to in the summer holidays, I was stunned to hear other students saying things like, 'Well, I did the obligatory three days with my parents and then made my escape.'

'Three days? Out of a six-week holiday?' I spluttered. 'You didn't want to be with your parents?'

It knocked me sideways to hear what they were saying, because when term ended I could not wait to get home to see mine!

Equally, I never, ever felt that I *had* to invite my parents to something, whereas for many of my friends that always seemed to be the case. There were events that you were meant to go to with parents and so they felt obliged to invite them, because their parents would be pissed off if they didn't go. But I always wanted my parents to come to things. It didn't cross my mind not to have them there.

When I left drama school, I focused on building a career. I fell in and out of love and had my heart broken; I got my Equity card, worked in live theatre and did a bit of television. At one point, I married the wrong man for the wrong reasons, got divorced and bounced back. It all seems like such a long time ago now! I think I took my parents' lead in getting through life's failures and disappointments: I relied on the comfort and support of friends and family; I picked myself up and carried on.

Like Mum and Dad, I was very sociable and always surrounded by friends. I was the girl at the party with a glass of wine in one hand, a fag in the other and a big smile on my face. Then I had Matthew and everything changed, but why? If you had put me in a line-up next to Joanne, my friend from drama school, who lived on her nerves and was highly neurotic and anxious, and if you had then asked people to pick out who would be most likely to suffer post-natal depression or anxiety, it would've been Joanne every time. But when Joanne had children, she had not a day of it, while I had it severely. There was no logic to it.

So, why me? Some people's depression starts because a spouse or a parent dies. For others, it is triggered by a nervous breakdown. Some people suffer an episode of depression because of financial worries and feeling overwhelmed. Others have no idea why they suffer depression; it's just because they are prone to it.

For me, it was having a baby – and having a baby is undoubtedly a traumatic experience. Whether it's a good experience or a bad one, it is a body trauma. But I often wonder: Had I not had a baby, would I never have experienced depression? Or would there have been something else in my life that brought it on? Was I always prone to it? Was there something inherent in me? Why didn't it manifest before I had a baby?

There are so many unanswered questions. Did having a baby open me up to living with depression for the rest of my life? Considering the high percentage of women whose life-long depression starts with having a baby, it seems that giving birth can be a massive trigger. Unfortunately, I was still a long way off finding out exactly why this was and what on earth to do about it.

IV

Even today, when it is so much easier to talk about mental illness, there are people who feel embarrassed about having depression. I was never embarrassed about it but, knowing how much my friends and family wanted me to bounce back to being bubbly Denise again, I tried to hide how I was feeling because I was so conscious that people wanted me to be well.

Although I remained in the grip of crippling depression, I started to pretend I was getting better. Tim used to walk into the house – as Lincoln does today, when I'm poorly – with a look of hope in his eyes. Had it lifted? Was I feeling better? It was upsetting to see how crushed he was when he realised the answer was no. It was tempting to force a smile and say, 'Do you know? I feel so much better,' and watch him light up.

None of my family put pressure on me to be well. They loved me too much to do that. But I put pressure on myself because I was aware of how my illness affected the way everybody else was feeling, especially my child, my husband and parents. I forced myself to try to be well in a way I would never have done if I were lying in bed with an obvious physical illness. If I'd been laid out with a neck brace and my legs in traction after a serious car accident, nobody would have let me get up and try to walk. Yet, because my depression was a mental illness and nobody could see it, some days I was doing the equivalent of running a marathon on two broken ankles, with cracked ribs and severe whiplash.

My sister, Debbie, was working on the cruise ships as a beauty therapist at the time. She came home after six months away thinking that seeing me and the baby was all going to be marvellous – and of course it wasn't. Debbie was very support-ive, bless her, but it was as much of a shock for her to see me as it was for everybody else. I had been so happy and carefree during my pregnancy.

If I'd had heart surgery or cancer, nobody would have ques-tioned that my recovery would be slow, but after a while I sensed that some of my friends were thinking, 'Come on, it must be getting better now. You've had it for five weeks!'

People don't like to be around people who are depressed, so my friends found it very difficult. Some of them stayed away, and I was glad they did, because often I didn't want to see anybody; I just wanted to curl up in a ball. Others said things like, 'Oh, you'll be fine. Let's go shopping and get you a new dress. That'll perk you up.'

It sounds like a lack of sympathy, but I understand where they were coming from. I was the person who made them feel better and it was disconcerting for them when that person disappeared. They wanted me to be well again – and I tried.

People of my granny's generation were the most unforgiv-ing. My granny loved me dearly, but her attitude was very much, 'Come on, pull yourself together.'

Her generation took a similar view to the GP I saw in London. They said things like, 'Well, we didn't have post-natal depression. We just had to get on with it.'

But if you asked, 'Whatever happened to Auntie Vera?' they would whisper, 'Oh, we don't talk about Vera. She went a bit funny after the birth and was never the same again. They had to put her away.'

Later, when I researched my illness in depth, I found that there was somebody of Granny's generation in every family who had 'gone a bit funny after the birth'. It's just that no one ever gave it a name.

My mum worked as a psychiatric nurse at Prudhoe Mental Hospital, as it was called then, a hospital near Newcastle for people with severe mental health disabilities. There was no doubt in Mum's mind that there were women in the hospital who, years before, had been put away for undiagnosed, untreated severe post-natal depression or puerperal psychosis, and that some of them eventually became institutionalised.

It is very scary to think that if I'd been born fifty years earlier, I could quite possibly have spent my life in an institution, instead of having all these wonderful years with my family, friends and career. Those poor women in Prudhoe Mental Hospital and elsewhere ended up being defined – and confined – by their mental illness, but I'm lucky enough to be in a position where it doesn't have to define me, and I won't let it.

While I was still at Mum and Dad's, Tim and I completed the sale on the Hemmel, our lovely house in Northumberland, the one we had fallen in love with during the pregnancy. It was only about eight miles from my parents' house, but I wasn't ready to move into it yet, although I knew I couldn't cling to Mum for ever. When we did move, a few weeks later, it was the freakiest time for me. I was already living in a surreal world, unable to feel emotion, with a baby I longed to love, and then suddenly we were in a new house.

Six weeks earlier, I had been a normal 31-year-old woman, happily pregnant, living in a flat in London, shopping for the baby at Brent Cross and looking forward to the future. Now I was only just managing to dress myself after weeks spent in my dressing gown, and the London flat had been swapped for a big house in the countryside that didn't feel like home. It was terrifying.

I was very unwell and confused. I really didn't know what was happening in my life. Fear of change is quite a common thread of mental illness – not just post-natal illness, but general depression and anxiety – and I think the move to the Hemmel sparked an enduring fear of change for me. I was desperate for my life to go back to how it had been before depression engulfed me. Instead each day brought further changes and trauma.

It was a terrible time for Tim. The partners of people with depression really suffer. Tim was over the moon about having a baby, but how could he enjoy his son while his wife was so poorly? And I was awful to live with, because I thought Tim was to blame for literally everything apart from my illness. Clutching at normality in my bizarre, surreal world, I needed everything to be just so and in its place. 'Why isn't this where it should be?' I'd screech at him. 'Why haven't you done this?'

My behaviour was completely irrational and yet Tim never criticised me or lost his patience. To let off steam, he would go in the garden and scream at the top of his lungs. Then he'd come back inside and try to be normal again, which must have been a mammoth effort because he was dealing with someone who felt no emotion, just panic, emptiness and dark-ness. It was particularly hard because he didn't know anyone else who had my illness. He didn't even know *of* anyone else who had it. Not only did neither of us have a point of refer-ence; nobody did, because my condition was hardly ever spoken about. You didn't go in a pub and hear someone say, 'My wife's suffering from depression,' whether it was post-natal or not.

Tim told me that when he did say something about it in the pub, people looked at him like he was crazy. 'What's she got to be depressed about?' they'd ask.

To the outside world, I had everything I could possibly want. I had a husband who loved me. I had a healthy child. I lived in this beautiful home in the countryside and I had money in the bank. Since people thought depression was circumstantial and that you only felt low if you had a reason to feel low – if you'd lost your job or if somebody you loved had died – they couldn't understand what could be wrong with me. And I don't resent them for it, because I understand. After all, until very recently, I had thought the same way.

They'd say to Tim, 'Oh, bloody Sam Murray's wife had a bairn a few weeks ago. She had a couple of weeks when she was mad as a bat, but she's fine now, man. Your wife'll get over it. She'll be champion. For God's sake, man, take her out to the Metrocentre and buy her something new. Cheer her bloody face up.'

'Yes, she'll be fine,' Tim used to say, although he didn't know if I would ever recover. None of us knew if I would get better. 'I felt like I'd lost my wife,' Tim told me, years afterwards. 'I was with this amazing woman, who was the life and soul of every party, who I loved and who desperately wanted a child. We got pregnant. She loved her pregnancy. We were so excited. And then I'd lost her. She was gone. The person I loved had gone.'

When I look back, I can see that although Tim was very supportive to me when I was poorly, my illness put a massive strain on our marriage. I don't think I understood how big a strain until, many years later, certain things came to light, when I realised that, although we'd been together twenty-four years, the rot had set in early on.

Even so, like Mum, Tim constantly reassured me – and that was my lifeline, because if you don't think you're going to get better, you start thinking, 'If this is life, it's not living. I can't go on like this.' And those kinds of thoughts lead to the tragic headlines.

I often sensed people thinking, 'Snap out of it, for God's sake,' so it made a world of difference that Tim knew I couldn't just snap out of it. However, he didn't see any harm in remind-ing me of the things that had mattered to me before depression overwhelmed me. A couple of weeks after we moved, he asked me to go and see a play with him at the Live Theatre Company in Newcastle. Live Theatre was – and still is – a vibrant, creative hub where Tim and I had both cut our teeth acting, and where Robson Green, Kevin Whately and Alun Armstrong all started out. We thought of ourselves as the Geordie mafia at Live Theatre.

I was reluctant to go, but Tim persuaded me. Sensing that he really wanted to go out, I left Matthew with my cousin, Kirsty. Matthew was only a tiny little thing and Kirsty was quite young and inexperienced, but I told myself that we weren't going to be gone for long. Three hours later, we walked back into the house to find Matthew crying hysterically and Kirsty looking like she'd had the worst night of her life. She had tried to swaddle Matthew and was rocking him on her shoulder, but he was crying to the point where he could hardly breathe.

'I'm so sorry! He's cried all night long. He's never stopped,' Kirsty wailed. 'I've tried him with a bottle. I've tried him with a dummy. Nothing's working.'

'Oh dear! Never mind, I'm here now,' I said, taking Matthew from her.

Matthew instantly stopped crying. Nestling into my shoulder, he went from hysteria to nothing, just like that.

'Wow,' I thought.

Suddenly there was a connection between us that I'd never felt before. That was the start of the good days and bad days, which is how the illness progressed: a few good days followed by bad days. It was still like being in a quagmire, but there were days when, I wouldn't say it had lifted, but it was not as severe as it could be – when the blackness turned grey.

The good days were never great, but they were better days, and I became slightly more functioning, although I was still going through the motions. I've got old VHS videos some-where showing visitors coming round to the new house and me out in the garden holding Matthew, looking to all intents and purposes like a really happy young mum, but feeling so lonely inside, and desperately unwell. There are photos too, from over the years, that show me smiling despite feeling poorly – and nobody would ever know, except me. It was just awful trying to get through those days.

I find it hard to look at the photos from Matthew's christen-ing in August 1989. I was wearing a striking red Cossack-style suit that day; I'd had hair extensions put in and liberally applied some red lipstick and blush – anything to zhoosh myself up a bit. I looked fine, but I remember spending the day in a grey fog, desperate for it to be over, longing for sleep. There were lots of people wanting photos of me and the baby, but I just wanted to lie down on my own in a room with the curtains closed. It was a big day, one of several really impor-tant days in my life that were ruined because of depression.

I didn't give a lot of thought to what was going to happen with my career. We were used to being a two-income family, but Tim didn't put pressure on me to go back to work, so I was more focused on how to treat my illness. Then, when Matthew was about four months old, Tim was driving me to Newcastle when Max Roberts, the director of Live Theatre, rang Tim's car phone. (Get Tim! He always told people that the first time I ever got into his car, I said, 'Eee, you've got a car phone!', which of course I didn't.)

Max Roberts was and continues to be a friend. He gave me one of my first jobs ever in the theatre, in the early eighties. He didn't know the depths of how poorly I had been, though. I might have said, 'I haven't been too grand lately,' but I didn't tell everyone.

Max explained that he was putting on a small-scale tour of a C.P. Taylor play, *And A Nightingale Sang*. It was showing at the Queen's Hall Theatre in Hexham and Val McLane, Jimmy Nail's sister, who was playing the mother – a leading role for an older actress – had slipped a disc and couldn't go on. In small productions, you don't have understudies. That only happens in commercial theatre, when the company has enough money to pay one. It was a crisis. 'Where are you? Could you come and read the part onstage?' Max asked.

I said yes.

I had no rehearsal time. I would be shown round the set when I arrived at the theatre, then when I got onstage I was to use my intuition. My instructions were to stay as still as possible while reading my lines from the book and let the other actors nudge me round the stage into the right blocking positions.

There was a lot of support there for me at the theatre. I knew everybody in the show because we were all the Geordie mafia. But, alone in my dressing room, as I put a Polaroid of Matthew up on the mirror, I started thinking, 'Oh my God, am I going to be able to do this?'

Thankfully, I wasn't ill that night. I was nervous, but I always am in theatre; there are very few actors who aren't. I was extremely nervous, though – it was worse than first-night nerves, as I was trying to create a performance within a couple of hours that the others had been creating over four weeks. I really didn't want to let anybody down.

Val is a much taller lady than me and, as she proudly tells everyone, she has size 9 feet, so I went round the theatre begging, stealing and borrowing what I could to get my costume together – a shawl here, a brooch there – and suddenly I was on, without even knowing what sort of voice I was going to use. I had to develop a character on the spot.

Somehow I got through it and received rapturous applause at the end. In a piece about how I'd stood in for Val at the last minute, the *Hexham Courant* wrote, 'Much to her surprise,

Denise did a fantastic job, and the majority of the audience thought that her character, a very religious woman, was carrying a Bible throughout the play!'

As an actress, that's a great compliment: I hadn't distracted from the piece, even though I didn't know my lines. People didn't realise that I was actually reading the script out loud; they thought I was performing using a Bible to reference how overzealous my character was!

It was a big boost for me as an actor to get a good review, but it was also a huge breakthrough for me as a person, after all that I'd been going through. A massive challenge had presented itself and I'd stepped up to meet it.

V

When Matthew was just under a year old, I was offered a part in *Byker Grove*, a BBC TV series for older kids set in a youth club in the Byker district of Newcastle. I was to play Polly, a tart with a heart and the mother of Donna, in eight or nine episodes. It was very exciting, as I hadn't done much television until then, but I couldn't help worrying about feeling poorly during filming. Although I was having fewer bad days, they were as grim as ever, and I knew it would be difficult to work through them.

I don't think there was ever a thought of turning the part down, though. Surviving the Live Theatre Company performance of *And A Nightingale Sang* had shown me that I was still able to work – and although I knew next to nothing about my illness and how it would progress, I was determined not to let it get in the way of my career.

Like buses, acting jobs tend to come all at once, so it shouldn't have been a surprise that around the same time Tim was offered a job in Australia filming a BBC TV series called *Boys From The Bush*. It was a starring role and a brilliant part, but there was a huge downside to taking it on: it meant that Tim would be filming in Australia for six months. Never mind. We decided that Matthew and I would join him once I had finished filming my episodes of *Byker Grove*.

Almost instantaneously, another job turned up; Jimmy Nail came round to the house and offered me a part in *Spender*, a BBC TV series he had written with my godfather, Ian La

Frenais. Honestly, what was going on? Was it something in the stars? I had no idea, except that Jimmy's offer presented me with a massive dilemma. If I took the part in *Spender*, I wouldn't be able to go to Australia with Tim; if I turned it down, I might never have another chance to star in a prestigious television drama.

In fact, I didn't really want to go to Australia. Not because I didn't want to be with Tim – I did – but because I was scared of being so far away from home and my comfort blanket. So although I knew that as a wife I should go to Australia, I decided to stay and do *Spender*, despite not really being well enough.

Tim and I didn't have the sort of marriage where the husband said, 'You've got to do this!' He gave his blessing for me to stay in the UK, but I realise now how hard it was for him to agree to it. He didn't want to spend six months away from us – and from Matthew, particularly – in a different time zone on the other side of the world. He'd be ringing us just before he went to bed, while Matthew and I were having our cornflakes. He was also worried about me taking on too much, because the filming schedules of *Spender* and *Byker Grove* were going to overlap for a few weeks, doubling my workload. Still, that's the way this business often works – feast or famine – and you either accept it or do something else for a career. We agreed that I would go to Australia as soon as the first series of *Spender* wrapped.

In the weeks that followed, I hated being away from Tim. I really missed him, especially on my bad days, because he was always so understanding when I was feeling poorly. Fortunately, I'm good at my job and was able to act my way through the bad days without anybody noticing. Life was very busy and the weeks sped past. In June, two months after we'd said goodbye, I had a fortnight off and the BBC very kindly paid for Matthew and me to fly business class to see Tim (it would never happen today!). Before I knew it, I was counting down the days to our flight to Australia – with a growing sense of trepidation, unfortunately.

I could never work out what brought on the bad days, if anything. There seemed to be no rhyme or reason to why the uninvited guest would visit. Years later, I found out that my illness is mainly endogenous, which means that most of the time it's not influenced by external factors. The visitor just turns up – and then he leaves again. He's unpredictable. Sometimes, though, I can feel myself drawing him closer, just by worrying that he will come, and as the date of my departure to Australia approached, I could feel him hovering nearby. The closer the day came, the worse I felt, until I was completely overwhelmed by anxiety at the thought of travelling so far away from home with my child.

The night before we left, I had a massive relapse into black depression. In hindsight, I probably should have cancelled the trip, but I didn't really feel I had a choice about going. The tickets were booked and I had to take Matthew to his father. So the next day I got on a Malaysia Airlines jumbo jet, with Matthew in my arms and an unwanted companion by my side.

Two weeks earlier, I had decided that I could manage a 24-hour journey with Matthew. I adored being a mum when I felt normal. I wasn't an organic, earth mother type – I was all for buying jars at the supermarket and there was never a terry nappy in sight – but I absolutely loved motherhood.

It felt as if the first year of having Matthew had been taken away from me, but now I was enjoying all the normal things about being a mother. When I went out for a walk with Matthew in his pushchair, I'd sometimes think, 'God, I'm a mum!' It was a bit of a delayed reaction, I think.

Matthew's first birthday was a joyous day. All my friends who had young babies came round, including Jimmy Nail's partner, Miriam Jones. My granny was there, my mum, and other family, and all these little bods were sat around the table with their little hats held on with elastic under their chins. 'Right, shall we sing "Happy Birthday"?' I said.

'Let me go and get the cake,' Miriam said.

'Whoops!' I said, because I'd forgotten all about getting a cake.

I can't put that down to depression. It was just me being hopeless. Miriam scooted off to the Co-op, bless her, and came back with a Thomas the Tank Engine cake, I think. Of course, my family weren't remotely fazed by this, but Miriam simply could not believe it.

'How could you forget a cake for your child's first birthday? You had one job!' she said.

Matthew's birthday had been a matter of weeks before, but it couldn't have felt more different from this. Taking him to Australia seemed an impossible task – especially as, on top of everything else, I had a paralysing fear of flying. I was the passenger who reaches out and squeezes the arm of the person in the next seat so tightly that it gives them a lasting bruise! I was the passenger who made involuntary yelping noises during mild turbulence. As the plane took off, I felt so scared and poorly that I wanted to die. Once we were in the air, I was in so much mental pain that I wouldn't have minded if the plane had plunged out of the sky and down into the sea.

It was horrendous. I felt I had to say something to the cabin staff. 'I'm not very well,' I explained, without going into detail, although I'm sure they could see it in my eyes.

The air stewardesses reacted with a level of sympathy and kindness that completely took me by surprise. As well as making sure I had everything I needed for the flight, they whisked Matthew off for four hours so that I could get some sleep. Matthew was thirteen months old and at that time his favourite toy was a little stick-on driving wheel. First they took him to the cockpit of the enormous jumbo jet and sat him down next to the captain for two hours. Next, they swept him up off to their private area at the back of the plane to look after him there. It was incredibly kind of them. I don't know what I would have done without them.

Somehow I got to the end of the journey, but I was in a really bad way when I stepped off the plane; my sense of unreality was off the scale. Australia felt a long way off even though I was actually there, and things were all the more bizarre because I had left England in a heatwave and was arriving in Melbourne on a grey winter's day.

Tim was at the airport to meet us with Mark Haddigan, his best friend out there. Mark played Tim's character's nephew in *Boys From The Bush*, and Mark's wife, Melanie, had arranged a little gathering to welcome us. Everyone was being so nice, but instead of going to a barbecue and celebrating our arrival, Tim had to take me straight to a psychiatrist to get some medicine to calm me down. It was a miserable start to what turned out to be a very tough trip.

Tim was staying in a newly built and newly decorated flat in the Melbourne suburb of Toorak. There's a particular smell of new carpet that I associate with that time and, like Ivoire by Balmain, my mother's perfume, it used to evoke a slight panic in me if I came across it in later years. It reminds me of the bleak hours I spent in the flat while Tim was working, desperately wishing I were back home in Northumberland. It felt so unfair. I was in a country I'd never visited before, surrounded by great people, but I couldn't enjoy myself at all.

Melanie was incredible with me, driving me here and there and taking the baby to give me a rest. But nothing was easy, and I was very aware that Tim wanted his wife back. He was worried about me, but the situation was deeply frustrating for him. So I did a lot of pretending. So much of my life at this point involved pretending, because everybody wanted me to be okay.

When the time came to go, I was torn. Much as I longed to get home, I didn't want to leave Tim. Then I got so ill again that I was too poorly to get on the flight home and Tim had to ring the BBC and say I wasn't well enough to do the journey. They were very understanding and offered to change the flight and rejig my filming schedule. This was in the days when television companies really looked after you, to the point that when Matthew and I finally landed at the airport in London, a few days later, there was a nurse waiting at the gate to accompany me back to Newcastle. She was in full uniform, mind, so it felt a lot like being met by Nurse Ratched from *One Flew Over the Cuckoo's Nest*! Still, I was grateful to her and to the BBC for their care and concern.

I am amazed that I managed that first trip to Australia, all things considered, but it really blows me away that I decided to go back, two months later, when I had another break in filming. Why on earth would I choose to go through the whole nightmare again? What was I thinking? This time, I decided to surprise Tim – partly because I love surprises, but also as a sort of insurance in case I suddenly couldn't go at the last minute. My reasoning was that if I was poorly and couldn't get on the plane, Tim would be none the wiser and so couldn't be disappointed. The only person I told was Melanie and she helped me to organise everything, knowing that I might not actually arrive.

Matthew was eighteen months old then and chattering away. Tim and I used to play this game with him where we'd point out someone famous on the news and tell him who it was. We found it hilarious that he could name several world leaders by the age of one and a half.

'Who's that?'

'Stormin' Norman!'

'Who's that?'

'John Major!'

He was so good on that second flight to Australia. When we stopped off in Kuala Lumpur, a man with grey hair and glasses came over to me in the business lounge and said, 'Your little boy is incredible.'

'Why? What did he say?' I asked.

'He just came over to me and asked, "Are you John Major?"'

Once we arrived in Melbourne, Melanie set up the surprise and Tim was absolutely thrilled to see Matthew and me again so soon. I was pleased that I'd braved the journey again, because this time it was a really nice trip, even though I had the occasional bad day. I felt very fortunate to be able to do the whole thing all over again and heal the memory of our first disastrous visit. I was also quite proud of myself that I had faced my fear and got on that plane, unwelcome guest be damned. It was a key moment in my long journey through this illness. I felt stronger afterwards and less afraid – and Mark and Melanie remain our best friends to this day.

VI

People often ask me, 'When did it get better?' The answer is that it didn't get better. It has lasted thirty years. There's no time limit.

But I guess I began to come through the worst of it around eighteen months after I had Matthew, which was when – for periods of time, at least – I started feeling more like the person I was before. I wasn't better, but sometimes I'd wake up in the morning and think, 'I feel normal.'

The 'normal' word is the most important word of all to anybody who's depressed. You're not longing for happiness, because it's not about being happy. It's about being normal. All you want is normality, and that includes having problems in your life. What you crave is the ability to deal with your normal life in a normal way, without depression.

Gradually, the number of normal days increased. I'd have five good days, two bad days, three good days and a bad day. There was no pattern to it, but over time the periods of wellness grew longer and the visitor stayed away.

In those days, I had an agent called Denis Beecher, who had been representing me since I'd left drama school. He was a bit like Steve Delaney's Count Arthur Strong – about 110 years old and slightly pompous. Thrilled that I was becoming known beyond the north-east, he'd become quite protective of my 'image'.

When our local paper in Newcastle, the *Evening Chronicle*, as it was then, requested an interview with me to talk about my role in *Spender*, I told Denis that I also intended to speak about my experience of post-natal depression.

'Well, that's a complete error of judgement in my opinion,' he said. 'They'll think you're mad, darling! Why on earth would you talk about such a thing? You'll never work again!'

I understand his reticence, because nobody else on TV was talking about this kind of thing. And while Denis thought it would destroy my career, my family were worried that I would be taking on too much by talking about it. But I made a decision then and there that if doing an interview about post-natal depression meant never working again, then so be it. If I could help other people going through it, I wasn't going to be put off by anything.

'I'm sorry, Denis, but I completely disagree with you,' I said. 'I can't imagine anybody going through what I did and not having the support I did, and I will speak out about it.'

The *Evening Chronicle* was the perfect springboard. Your local paper always championed you if you were doing something a little bit different, and I had been on their radar since I was eighteen and went to drama school, when they published a photo of me peering out from behind a tree above a caption saying something like, 'Local lass goes to drama school to hit the heights of showbiz!'

Obviously they were going to ask me to do an interview when *Spender* and *Byker Grove* were broadcast; and during the interview, I knew, they were likely to ask me about being a working mum. So I told the journalist a story about how Matthew had played the part of 'Baby Edward' in an episode of *Spender* and had cried throughout his scenes. 'I had to keep giving him an endless supply of Gold Bar biscuits to suck on to try and keep him quiet.' I laughed.

'But I've been very poorly,' I told her, and she was incredibly interested to hear about my illness, and wrote it up sympathetically in her article.

The next thing I knew, *Woman's Own* got in touch – back when *Woman's Own* was a nice magazine that featured knitting patterns and Roger Moore on the front cover – and asked if I would do a feature on post-natal depression for them. I was surprised, as I was an avid magazine reader and yet I had never read anything about mental illness or post-natal depression in the weeklies or monthlies. (I remember finding a book about depression in the library, but the post-natal depression section inside it was tiny. There were a few dusty old journals, but nothing up to date.)

The *Woman's Own* piece led to invitations to appear on audience participation shows like *Kilroy* with Robert Kilroy-Silk and *The Time, The Place* with John Stapleton. This wasn't because I was famous, as I was only just becoming known; it was because nobody else was talking about it.

There was always a mix of people on these shows, so as well as giving me a platform to speak about post-natal depression, it was interesting for me to meet the other guests. I was always looking for someone who had post-natal depression as badly as I had it and vividly remember meeting someone who'd had severe puerperal psychosis. I told her all about Tim's changing moustache, and looking down at Matthew and thinking, 'Why have I got this baby here?'

It was nothing compared to what this woman had been through with her psychosis. She'd literally had no idea who she was and had thought that her child was possessed by the devil. It made me thankful that I hadn't had it, after all – even though, with the right treatment, she had gone on to make a full recovery.

I also liked meeting the guest 'experts' on these talk shows, even if I didn't always agree with them. I'll never forget the psychologist I met on an episode of *The Time, The Place* about post-natal illness.

'What a shame that you were poorly,' she said to me. 'But I would have been able to spot that you were prone to post-natal depression when you were pregnant.'

'Actually, in my case, you wouldn't,' I said.

'I'm a trained psychologist and I would have been able to tell,' she insisted.

By then I had started to hear from other people about their illness, and they had listed the indicators of post-natal depression during their pregnancies, which included feeling sad, irritable, angry, hopeless and worthless. I'd had none of those symptoms. I had also met a woman who suffered from pre-natal depression and then went on to be fine once her baby was born (and I've since met several others like her.)

'I'm not disputing that you're highly qualified in your field, but I beg to differ,' I told the psychologist. 'I was the typical blooming woman in pregnancy. I was the exception to the rule – if there is a rule.'

One of the other guests on this particular show was a lady called Dr Katharina Dalton, a British physician who had coined the phrase 'premenstrual syndrome' in 1953 after researching hormone levels in women during their menstrual cycle, and later came up with the term 'post-natal depression'. These illnesses had been going on since the dinosaurs, but were only given names in the twentieth century! It shows you just how little consideration was given to new mothers by the medical profession, historically.

Dr Dalton made her breakthrough after she became pregnant for the first time and noticed that her monthly premenstrual headaches had disappeared. She put this down to the natural increase in progesterone during pregnancy and began successfully treating PMS sufferers with progesterone. Subsequently, she linked post-natal depression with the natural drop in progesterone after giving birth and treated it in a similar way to PMS.

She was on the programme to talk about how she had intervened in the case of a woman called Anna Reynolds, who at the age of seventeen had killed her mother as a result of having severe post-natal illness. After Reynolds went to prison for life, Dr Dalton managed to have her sentence revoked and get her released from jail by proving that her actions had been triggered by an extreme imbalance in her hormones.

Dr Dalton's theories made sense to me. She had come up against a lot of resistance from her male colleagues in the 1950s when she argued that symptoms of PMS, like headaches, fatigue, irritability and depression, were more physical than psychological. My experience completely chimed with her theory. My life had been blissfully happy until I'd plunged into a black, thick depression just after having a baby, so I knew my illness didn't stem from a psychological problem. Yes, it was affecting my brain and consequently my mind, but that's not where the problem originated, however many doctors tried to blame it on bogus psychological issues.

After meeting Dr Dalton on *The Time, The Place*, I went to my local GP and said, 'You need to treat me with progesterone.'

'Okay. I don't know how to do that,' he said.

So I arranged for Dr Dalton to liaise with my doctor and treat me with progesterone, although unfortunately it didn't go on to have the desired effect. Almost twenty years later, I discovered that she had been right about the hormone imbalance but not about the hormone. It was one of many avenues that turned out to be dead ends in my search for effective treatment, and it's very frustrating to think about how close I came to the answer.

There was no social media in those days, and no access to online information. People had to write to you if they wanted to respond to something you had said in the press or on television. As one of the first 'personalities' to speak openly about post-natal illness, I received lots of letters on the subject, including a pamphlet from a post-natal illness group based in the Lake District, which they sent me after seeing *The Time, The Place*.

Like the association I had contacted nearly two years earlier, this group sent out literature aimed at sufferers of post-natal depression. But this time, as I looked down the list of symptoms associated with post-natal depression in their pamphlet, I felt at last that I had found someone who understood what I'd been going through. For the first time ever, written down in black and white, I saw the words, 'A childlike desire for one's mum', which was among the more obscure symptoms of my illness.

It was a massive moment for me. I had beaten myself up for my childlike desire for my mum; I had told myself I was being weak and pathetic. 'What if I didn't have a mum?' I used to ask myself. 'What about people who haven't got a mum?'

But here it was, a symptom of my illness, not a deep-rooted issue from childhood, or a reason for self-flagellation. Other people with post-natal depression had exactly the same feelings! I wasn't the only one. Just the simple fact of seeing it written down was a huge help to me.

It was a real breakthrough, because I had felt so isolated for so long. Now at last I had people to talk to who really understood my suffering. I wrote to the group and was put in touch with a couple of people who I spoke to on the phone, which was helpful. I tended to find myself in the comforting role, rather than the comforted, but it was still good to make contact.

As more and more people started approaching me to talk about post-natal depression, I realised how crucial it was that someone was speaking out about it. 'This might sound silly,' one woman told me, 'but I suffer from the same illness as you and I sleep with your cuttings by my bed, in case I need to read them in the middle of the night and remind myself that I'm not alone.'

Years later, after I had talked about post-natal depression on *Lorraine* one day, I had a letter from a guy who said, 'You saved my wife's life.'

It sounds very dramatic, but his wife was very poorly, and while I was talking about how poorly I had been, he yelled, 'Look at this Denise Welch. Look, look, look!'

In the depth of her misery and fog and depression, his wife looked up and saw me, a healthy woman (at that point), who had a child and a successful career, talking about my illness – her illness.

It gave her hope that she would get better – and that's what you need when you're as poorly as she was. 'She turned a corner that day,' her husband wrote.

These women's stories are the reason why I made it my mission to speak out about my experience of post-natal illness and how, for me, it developed into a lifetime of living with clinical depression. I am writing this book for them and anyone else who has suffered from anxiety and depression.

PART 2

Depression

I

There are several ways my illness can manifest. The unwelcome visitor can arrive any time and any how. He can come overnight, without any warning, without it crossing my mind that he might be on his way: I'll have dinner with a good friend, go to bed, watch one of my favourite rubbish reality shows on TV, fall asleep and when I wake up in the morning, he's there.

He comes unexpectedly during the day, too, even at life's happiest moments. I can be sitting on a beach in the sunshine, enjoying my holiday, with waves lapping over my feet; then suddenly the colour drains from my world and, whoosh, he's arrived.

Sometimes he comes wearing a very black cloak. Other times, his cloak is grey and I can sense him hovering nearby; or he knocks on the door, but doesn't come in. My depression is milder on the days he wears his grey cloak, but it's just as dangerous as on the days when he's wearing black. Mild depression is almost worse than severe depression because it doesn't stop you in your tracks: you just keep going, feeling awful, wondering if the pain will ever end.

Sometimes there are warning signs that the unwelcome visitor is coming, but I won't be aware of them until afterwards, when I look back and realise that I've been worrying about things that don't usually bother me, or trying to pack so much into my life that I end up feeling overwhelmed. It's hard to know which comes first, the chicken or the egg: is anxiety part of the progression of my illness, or does my natural tendency to worry push me over the edge into depression during times of stress? Possibly, it's a bit of both, depending on the situation.

After living with depression for three decades, I'm more in control of the beast, sometimes; but when it comes on endogenously and enters my system, there is nothing I can do about it, apart from clear my diary and go to bed. Of course, that's not something I have the luxury of doing when I'm working. Then I have to face the fear of going onstage or in front of the camera feeling poorly.

On a normal day, every actor worries about not being good and messing up their lines. It's an awful feeling, but it's ten times worse with depression, when your brain is befuddled and it's hard to remember anything. The only way to cope is to let go of the fear, something I discovered quite early on in my illness when I was doing a run of a play about football called *The Beautiful Game* at the Theatre Royal in Newcastle.

The play was really fun and had been going well up until then, but one afternoon my illness suddenly came on and I felt too poorly and too scared to go to work. By six o'clock in the evening, I was in the conservatory at the Hemmel wearing a pink kimono-type dressing gown, with the unwelcome visitor sitting opposite me. It was time for me to leave for the theatre – in fact, I should have been dressed, out the door and on my way – but I was feeling so bad that I couldn't motivate myself to get ready. Tim was away filming. Matthew was at my mum and dad's. I was alone in the house, paralysed by fear and depression.

Jimmy Nail happened to be passing by just then, on his way back from filming somewhere, and on the off-chance dropped in to say hello. I'd known Jimmy for a while and had been playing his character's ex-wife in *Spender*.

'Is everything all right?' he asked when he saw me in my dressing gown.

'I can't go to the theatre! I've got my depression,' I told him. 'What am I going to do?'

Jimmy frowned. 'What's the worst that can happen?' he said gently. 'You're on the stage, you can't carry on and you run off – and the next day there's a story in the *Evening Chronicle* saying, "Denise Welch had a panic attack and ran offstage during the show".' He shrugged. 'Nobody will die.'

It was exactly what I needed to hear, but I don't imagine to this day Jimmy realises what a huge effect his words had on me. He was probably just thinking, 'Bloody hell, I don't know why I popped in here with this mad woman! What can I say just to get out the door?'

So it's quite comical to think that as I go along in life dealing with depression, picking up helpful soundbites and mantras along the way, one of my favourites is, 'What's the worst that can happen?' – and 'Nobody will die' is another.

Jimmy's words of advice helped a lot and I was able to go onstage that evening. But whenever I got an acting job after that, my first thought was always, 'Oh God, what if I get ill?'

My illness was, and still is, a consideration in my work, especially so in those early days. So I experienced a sense of dread as well as elation when I was offered the lead in the C.P. Taylor play, *And A Nightingale Sang*, at the Newcastle Playhouse, a prestigious repertory company in my home town. This was the same play I had read through onstage at the Queen's Theatre in Hexham, when Matthew was four months old and I'd stepped in for Val McLane after she'd slipped a disc. Two years later, in 1991, I was playing Helen, the disabled sister, a major role that had a lot of lines and monologues.

I decided I was well enough to take it on.

The cast was fantastic. Val McLane was playing the mother again and Angie Lonsdale was playing my sister. It was the first time I had met Angie and she went on to become one of my best friends. Also starring were Robson Green, Davey Whitaker and Donald McBride, all stalwarts of the Geordie acting mafia. Meanwhile, Ian Sharrock, who at the time was married to my great friend Pam, had just come out of *Emmerdale* and wanted to do some theatre, so I asked the play's director, Alan Lydiard, if he could audition Ian for the role of my character's boyfriend.

Ian was from Yorkshire and I gave him a crash course in how to do a Geordie accent, including key phrases to repeat to himself when he was alone. It always made me laugh when I was onstage and caught sight of him in the wings pacing up and down before his entrance, muttering, 'Stick a rubber hose up your nose, you big fat fucker,' over and over again.

Years later, while I was interviewing Britney Spears, I was rehearsing for 'Steel Magnolias' and asked her to listen to my Louisiana accent. I then asked her to say a non-sweary version of this phrase. Let me just say, I was much better than her . . .

The rehearsals period for *And A Nightingale Sang* was quite stressful for me because the director and I were on different pages. I'm not a method actress – I work instinctively, according to how I feel inside – and I felt he kept trying to go against that. I was quite forthright about my views, which added to my first-night nerves because I wanted to prove I was right, so it was a relief when we got fantastic reviews and tickets started selling out. I felt my stance had been justified.

My drinking started to gather momentum during this time, although I was never a daytime drinker and I have never, ever in my life had a drink before a show. I know people who do drink before shows, and people who have gone on drunk and given an amazing performance, unbelievably. I never was that person – but after the show, I would drink.

There was a wine bar on Grey Street in Newcastle that used to have a late-night licence. The local pubs rang the bell for last orders at 10.30 p.m. or 11 p.m. – around the time we were coming offstage – but the Grey Street wine bar had a downstairs area that was open until about midnight. We all used to go to drink and dance there. We had some really fun times. 'Summer Breeze' by the Isley Brothers reminds me of those nights; Robson and I loved that song.

One night, I drank too much red wine and woke up the next day with a stonking hangover, feeling really poorly and ill. I was angry with myself because my hangovers were always terrible – I was never somebody who bounced back by lunchtime – and with a hangover came mild depression and the fear that it would get worse.

My mind began to spin and I started beating myself up. 'Oh no, what have I done? How could I be so stupid? I'm going to feel terrible tonight.'

When I remembered that we had a matinee as well as an evening performance that day, the full 'hangxiety', as it is now known, kicked in. I started to panic and think: 'How am I going to get through? What if I can't remember my lines? What if I run offstage?'

Everybody else was fine when I went into work. They were saying the kinds of things normal people say after tying one on the night before: 'Oh God, I feel like shit. Do you? Wish I hadn't had that extra bloody glass. Anyway, let's get through these shows and then we can go again. Hahaha.'

Listening to them, all I could think was, 'This is terrible, absolutely terrible.'

It took every ounce of determination in my body to force myself to go on for the matinee performance, but I was soon wishing I hadn't. Alone on the stage, in the middle of a monologue, I felt black depression starting to whoosh through me, from my toes upwards. It was like being in a nightmare: I was engulfed in blackness, standing in front of an auditorium full of people, trying to remember my lines.

Gripped by panic, I kept thinking, 'I can't stand it. I'm going to run off!'

All the while, the words of the play were coming out of my mouth, as if nothing was wrong.

Somehow I managed to stay onstage until the interval. When I came off I collapsed in a chair with my head in my hands. 'Are you all right, darling?' Ian and Robson asked.

'I wish I had cancer,' I blurted out.

They were appalled. 'What are you talking about?' they said.

'If I had cancer, I'd come off and say, "I've got cancer, and I feel terrible," and you guys wouldn't let me go back onstage.'

They looked bemused. 'Oh, you'll be fine, Den. Howay, man,' they said. 'You got through the first half. Go on, you're brilliant.'

They weren't being unsympathetic – they were my friends – but they couldn't understand what was wrong, because I'd just given a great performance, despite everything. Often, people don't have the slightest sense of what I'm going through, because they can't see it and don't know much about depression and mental illness.

Some of my friends have flown off the handle when I've told them this story. 'If you knew how awful cancer was, you wouldn't say such a thing!' they say.

Cancer is a word that lights a touchpaper for many people, especially if they have lost a loved one to this horrendous disease, and it goes without saying I wouldn't want actually to be afflicted by it. My point was that while people know that cancer is a severe physical illness and understand how serious it is, they don't understand how serious depression is, and I wish they did, because there would be a lot more sympathy for sufferers.

Of course I went back on after the interval, and also did the evening performance later. I had to: there was nobody to take my place. But I couldn't wait to have a glass of wine after the second show. 'I got through it! Now I need a drink,' I thought.

If I had to pick the pivotal moment when I started drinking to suppress the pain of my illness, that might well be it.

After the Newcastle run, we took the play to Edinburgh, where I shared a flat with Robson and Ian. Tim was away in Australia again, filming the second series of *Boys From The Bush*, and my sister was looking after Matthew.

One day, Angie and I went shopping on the Royal Mile and bought Matthew a sweet little Scottish tam-o-'shanter and tartan dungarees. I know I wasn't well because I can clearly remember what I was thinking as I was choosing this little outfit. My thoughts were see-sawing between worrying about being away from Matthew and feeling quite glad that I didn't have the responsibility of looking after him, in case I got poorly and wanted to be on my own. Back and forth they swung, between anxiety and relief, in quite a weird way.

Although I was teetering on the edge of depression, we still had some good times up in Edinburgh. None of us was famous, but Robson had been in *Casualty*, and if we couldn't get into a nightclub, he would say something mad to the bouncers, like, 'But you must remember me from *Casualty*! Jimmy the porter?'

He would do an impression of jauntily pushing a wheel-chair along, singing the *Casualty* theme tune.

'No, get lost,' the bouncers would say. 'You're not coming in.'

Pam came up to stay with us during the run and one night we were up late talking about who we would fancy if we weren't married. Suddenly, we heard a loud rap at the door.

Pam opened the door to a very angry woman, who strode into the flat, pointed randomly at Robson, and said, 'I live upstairs. I work in a caring profession and I'm trying to get some sleep. I don't give a shit if you'd shag Goldie Hawn. Can you just shut up?'

The next day, my friend Melanie Haddigan came up to stay; well, you know what they say, the more, the merrier! But unfortunately for Melanie, who had come to have fun with her actress friend, I came down with a bug the next morning. I was really physically poorly: feverish, sweating cobs and throwing up.

Melanie and Pam looked after me, bless them. 'Are you going to be able to go on tonight?' Melanie asked worriedly.

'I have to go on,' I croaked.

I didn't have an understudy, so it didn't enter my head that I couldn't perform, no matter what was wrong with me. We were on at one of the big Edinburgh theatres, too: not a fringe venue, but a proper theatre. The show had to go on.

After a few hours of fevered sweating and being sick, I started to feel my depression coming on. Delirium was causing a detachment between me and real life, and I had that familiar feeling of being in a dream sequence. I didn't tell anyone, though. They were being enough of a godsend just helping me out with my physical symptoms.

I got through the show and afterwards the girls took me home, put me to bed with cold flannels on my head and tried to persuade me to eat something. 'You were brilliant,' Melanie said. 'I would have never known you were ill!' (She meant physically poorly.)

The next day I couldn't remember anything about the night before. Not a thing about being onstage or coming home. It was as if someone had taken a pair of scissors and cut it out of my memory. I was terrified of doing theatre after that.

Nowadays, when I'm up for a theatre job and worrying about getting ill, I remind myself that live theatre is always very scary – and first-night nerves can be off the scale. On the first night of a play, every single actor in the world stands backstage, asking themselves, 'Why did I accept this job? I could have said no! Why did I say yes? What if I dry? Why do I put myself through this?'

It's absolutely awful, and far worse combined with depression, so I can totally understand why Stephen Fry did a runner in the middle of a West End play, a few years after I was up in Edinburgh. He obviously had a massive episode of depression and couldn't go back on at the interval, so he left the theatre, jumped on a ferry to Bruges and never returned. He was panned for it afterwards, but I felt nothing but sympathy.

I've been onstage with the unwelcome visitor on many a night. It still happens today: he will be with me as I am waiting to go on and I'll be silently screaming at him to go away.

'I have no choice but to go on and do this, you fucker,' I shout at him. 'You being here isn't going to stop me: I'm going to do it with or without you, so you may as well just fuck off!'

I still use Jimmy's mantra and think to myself: 'What's the worst that can happen? If I run off, nobody will die.'

Just in case I need to make a dash for it out of the theatre, I always know my exact route to the stage door. I've never done it (although I'm amazed I haven't) and hopefully never will, but I need to know which way I'll go, because you never know.

People might think depression is a weakness. Sometimes I have to remind myself that the fact that we're still here and can still do these things means that our tribe is very, very strong.

II

In the early stages of my illness, I lived in hope that one day it would go away for good. When I had a really good space of wellness, every single day I'd think, 'Maybe it's not coming back!'

So when it did come back, it would destroy me, and I grew very fearful of the visitor's sudden appearances. Sometimes I felt he was stalking me; other times I seemed to draw him to me simply by worrying that he might come.

It still happens today, very occasionally. 'Wouldn't it be awful if he came now?' I think, and my heart begins to race, my hands tingle and I get a tinny taste in my mouth. And then he arrives, sometimes within days or hours, often within seconds.

The first time it happened, Tim and I had booked a holiday in the sun with our friends Paul and Linda Squire. We were going to Tenerife, two couples, without children, and we were all looking forward to it, especially Linda, who didn't often get opportunities to be away from her children and was cock-a-hoop at the thought of the relaxing week ahead.

The trip was all booked and paid for. It was just a small, cheap-as-chips holiday, but nevertheless we'd been talking excitedly about it for weeks. Linda and I were very close then and still are – I'm godmother to her son, Jamie – and it made me happy to see how thrilled she was. Then a horrible thought entered my head, about a fortnight before we were leaving: 'Wouldn't it be awful if I got ill when we were on holiday with Linda and Paul?'

My heart began to beat rapidly. 'Especially as Linda is so excited about this trip,' my thoughts raced on. I tried to put it out of my mind.

In the week that followed, I filled up my days so that I didn't have time to overthink things, because my anxiety would set my heart pounding. However, before long, I felt myself getting ill. It was dreadful. Our departure date was imminent and I couldn't do anything about it.

About a week before we left, Tim was away somewhere filming and Linda rang for a chat. 'What are you going to wear on the journey?' she asked eagerly. 'What are you taking in your suitcase?'

The worry that my depression was going to ruin Linda's holiday set my heart racing again. I felt my illness coming on and, when I got off the phone, the cloud of depression that engulfed me was so thick and so bad that I had to call a friend to come and take Matthew for me.

Late that evening, alone in the house, I started to feel pins and needles all through my body. My hands tensed up and I couldn't move my fingers; my mouth twisted to one side and I couldn't speak. I had no idea what was happening; my body was out of my control. It was probably one of the most terrifying moments of my life.

I decided that I had to get to my parents. Although I could barely hold the steering wheel, I got into my car and drove the eight miles to Ebchester. My mum took one look at me and called the doctor, who came out, even though it was around midnight. (It was in the days when doctors came out at all hours, but I'm not sure I'd like to try it nowadays.)

When the doctor arrived, I was sitting on the sofa, my mouth twisted, my hands locked. He examined me and then stepped out of the room to speak to my mum.

'This is an extreme case of depression, *extreme*,' he told her.

He came back into the lounge and held my frozen hands in his. 'We may have to take you in for electroconvulsive therapy,' he said.

Just then Tim arrived in a fluster, having got home to find the house empty and rung my parents to ask where I was. Although I could hardly speak because my lips were so contorted, I managed to say, 'I can't go on the holiday. You've got to tell them I can't go.'

'Don't worry about the holiday!' my mum said, for the hundredth time. 'Let's focus on getting you better.'

'The holiday doesn't matter at all, pet,' Tim echoed.

I gave him a beseeching look. 'You've got to tell them,' I pleaded.

He nodded. 'Right, I will.'

He went to the phone in the hall, picked up the receiver and rang the Squires. When he came back, he said, 'It's all sorted. Linda's going to take a friend. She's absolutely champion and she says, "Get well soon".'

At that, my hands started to unlock and my mouth untwisted. All I needed was to know that I wasn't going to be responsible for ruining somebody else's holiday.

The doctor didn't take me in for electroconvulsive therapy (ECT) because I began to improve while he was still there, but there's no doubt that my depression was so bad that ECT was the next step, which shows how poorly I was. It was frightening to think that mental illness could have such an extreme physical effect. My facial paralysis was similar to Bell's palsy; I had never imagined that my mind could have so much power.

Anybody who has ever had butterflies in their tummy knows what it is like to experience the power of mind over body. It's that feeling you get when you're waiting to go in for an exam or do your driving test, give a presentation at work or go onstage. Some people get so nervous that they vomit; others start sweating and trembling, or come out in a rash. All of these physical symptoms start in the mind.

Although it was never as bad again, the night my hands froze opened me up to the fear of being able to bring on my illness just by worrying about it. Since then, I've had to train myself not to think, 'Wouldn't it be awful . . . ?', in case just the fear of the fear sets my heart racing.

I seem to be at my most vulnerable when my eyes are closed and I'm having a massage or sitting in a make-up chair. Then, if I'm not careful, I think about the visitor and my heart starts up; I can almost feel the whoosh before it comes. I've jumped off a lot of massage tables pretending I was feeling sick, panicked that my thoughts will upset my body chemistry and bring on an episode of depression.

Sometimes my body muddles up panic and excitement, with the same upsetting outcome. It happened just before I was due to sing 'It's Raining Men' with Coleen Nolan on the lunchtime talk show, *Loose Women*, about fifteen years ago. I was nervous that day – after all, it's quite something to sing on live television with one of the Nolans, dressed in galoshes and a yellow mac – but I was also thinking, 'What a fun thing to do!'

I arrived at the ITV studios feeling excited. However, as I sat in the make-up chair and closed my eyes to have my eyeshadow applied, the unwelcome visitor must have thought, 'Ooh, she's in make-up! I'm just going to pop along there.'

I probably had a hunch that he was coming, because I thought, 'Wouldn't it be awful if he came now?'

A moment later, I sensed him nearby and my heart started racing.

'Sorry, I feel a bit sick,' I told the make-up artist. 'Do you mind if I take a second? I need some air.'

I left the room and paced up and down the corridor outside, full of dread. 'He's coming . . . he's coming,' I thought.

In a trice he was on me, sucking all the fun and excitement out of the day. After that, I had no choice but to go on and perform the song with Coleen, wrapped in a thick cloud of depression. Yet, anybody who knew I had depression that day and saw me singing away on TV would have thought, 'Come on, it can't be that bad.'

I get it all the time. A friend will call and ask, 'How are you feeling?'

'I still feel really bad,' I'll say.

'Well, you looked fine on telly today!' they'll exclaim.

I want to yell, 'Of course I looked fine on telly today, because that's the mask that most of us with depression have to wear, especially in the public eye!'

This aspect of the illness can be very difficult for a partner to cope with. Sometimes, if a friend phones up, my voice will go into 'pretendy mode' as I try to appear completely fine. Then my partner (once Tim, now Lincoln) walks in and as I put down the phone, the mask switches from smiling to tragic. So it's not surprising if he complains, 'But you're fine when you're talking to Sue and I get this face!'

We feel we don't have to keep up the pretence with our partners, and ultimately they understand that. At the same time, they so desperately want us to be well. They want the person who's on telly or talking to Sue.

Although I have made the lifestyle changes I needed to make to minimise my depression, I still get slightly worried when I'm looking forward to something, because there's always a whisper in my mind saying, 'Wouldn't it be awful . . .'

Just last year, I texted my husband, Lincoln, before our holiday, to say, 'I'm really excited about going to Barbados, just you and I, for a fortnight on our own.'

As I tapped out the message, I felt a flip in my tummy, as the visitor edged a little closer and said, 'I'm always here, you know.'

Then he was gone.

That's me now, thirty years on, whereas years ago, I might have said, 'I'm excited' about something, and he would have said, 'Are you, now? Because I might just pay you a little visit.'

And my heart would pound as I felt him coming closer and closer.

I'm not really sure what is happening inside my body when the unwelcome visitor pays a call. What I do know is that depression is caused by a chemical or hormonal change in your system. Whether reactively or endogenously, something happens to stop the serotonin going to your brain. Serotonin is a chemical that affects many different functions of the body, including appetite, sexual desire and sleep, but is best known for its role in mental well-being and happiness.

Serotonin levels are affected when the adrenal glands release adrenaline combined with too much cortisol. Cortisol is a hormone that controls many important functions, including emotional responses, mood regulation, sleep, memory and, crucially, the body's fight-or-flight response to stress or danger. Too much of it upsets the balance of these functions.

Why does it happen, though? Does my dread of getting ill start my heart racing, which then triggers a flood of cortisol in my body, messing up my brain chemistry? Somehow it makes sense that a stressful thought can spark my perhaps overactive and ultra-sensitive fight-or-flight response.

What I don't understand is how I can be in the middle of a conversation with a friend, or in a shop buying a harmless stick of mascara, feeling fine – not nervous, not anxious, without a thought for my illness – and suddenly I get the tinny taste in my mouth, my hands tingle and everything changes. Why would my brain start releasing cortisol then?

While we wait for scientific advances in the understanding of mental illness, it's helpful simply to know that depressive illness is caused by chemical imbalance. That's basically it: chemical imbalance, which causes all illnesses. Cancer is chemical imbalance and so is depression. Knowing this, I am a huge advocate of antidepressant drugs, which work by replacing chemicals in your body that are depleted or missing, including serotonin. I'm pretty sure I wouldn't be here today without them.

III

Most people associate depression with circumstance. Those who don't suffer from it as an illness draw from their own experience of being depressed for circumstantial reasons, like a break-up, a bereavement or financial worries.

People get 'depressed' because they're going bankrupt and their world has turned upside down, but if suddenly they get a cheque for £100,000, their depression will go. Theirs is not depressive illness; it's feeling traumatised. It's all of the other words that describe mental suffering, and can be every bit as hard, but it's not depressive illness, for which there is often no reason or explanation.

It works the other way, too. During traumatic times, you might expect someone who suffers from clinical depression to have an episode of illness. Yet, when Mum was diagnosed with cancer in 1991, although my sister, Debbie, and I were devastated by the thought that we might lose our beloved mum, my unwelcome visitor stayed away.

Mum's diagnosis was a terrible shock for all of us, because she wasn't showing any signs of illness at all. It was her dentist who suspected something was up, after he discovered a white spot at the back of her throat.

When he commented on it, Mum said, 'Oh, I'm glad you've mentioned that. I've been feeling like I've got a bit of apple stuck there.'

He sent her for tests and that was it: cancer of the soft palate. If she hadn't gone to the dentist, I think she would have put up with it as something mildly irritating she had to live with. That was Mum: we always used to laugh that when she had a cold, nobody had ever been as poorly as she was, but when she had something really serious wrong with her, she said she felt completely fine.

The next couple of months were horrendous. Mum had to endure six weeks of agonising radiotherapy treatment and her mouth filled up with so many ulcers that she couldn't eat. I was incredibly worried about her. I hated to see her suffering. And yet I stayed well.

Mum got through her treatment and made a good recovery, with her sense of humour intact, bless her. About a year later, however, her doctors discovered a secondary oral cancer and she was faced with a very difficult choice. She had two options: radical, life-changing surgery that would most likely result in disability, or six months to live.

Mum went with Dad to see the doctors to discuss what to do. Back at the house, Debbie and I sat drinking brandy, like people in the movies do when they're waiting for bad news. Fearing the worst, I tried to take solace in the thought that Mum had at least seen her first grandchild, three-year-old Matthew, whom she worshipped and adored. I felt very sad, but not clinically depressed.

When Mum and Dad got back from the hospital, we all played cards together, which was slightly weird, as we hadn't played cards together in years. Meanwhile, Mum explained that her operation would involve removing two-thirds of her soft palate, the soft tissue at the back of the roof of the mouth that plays an important part in swallowing, breathing and speaking. To replace it, the surgeon would pull matching tissue down from the temple. This would leave a big indentation in Mum's head and she might never be able to talk again or swallow properly. There was also a chance that she might be on a drip for life. She was fifty-five.

Mum's mind was made up. 'I can't go through that,' she said. 'I've had a really good innings. I've got two wonderful daughters. I've seen my grandson born. I'd rather go out with a fag and a glass of whisky at a party than end up like that.'

Debbie and I were incredibly upset, but when Mum and Dad had gone to bed, we talked about how we had to accept Mum's decision; however difficult it was, we had to understand and respect it. I was very thankful that night to have a sibling.

Fortunately, Mum's doctors persuaded her to talk to someone else who had undergone the operation. Since it was quite a rare form of surgery, she had to travel to Sunderland to meet them; a man in his seventies, who had survived it and thrived. After speaking to him, Mum had a think and changed her mind: she decided that she was going to go through with the procedure after all.

Never once in the weeks building up to Mum's surgery, with all the doubts and fears that came with it, did I get my illness. The thirteen hours that Mum was in theatre were horrifically tense. I was worried and stressed in the same way that my sister and father were, but I didn't have an episode of depression.

When Mum came round from the operation, we almost couldn't bear to go in and see her. We didn't know what to expect. Had we lost the mum we knew? Had she lost herself? The tension was almost unbearable, and yet my reactions throughout were normal reactions to a traumatic situation. This is what I crave when I'm poorly: the ability to feel, whether it be to feel sad while Mum was suffering, or happy when she started getting better and began speaking again, against the odds. I'm pleased to say that she was back to her glamorous, 'Joan Collins' self within months and went on to see four more grandchildren born, which astounded her doctors.

Had I had depression while all of this was happening, it would have been terrible, not just for me, but for my mum, dad and sister, too. While Mum was ill and needed her loved ones around her, I simply wanted to feel the same way everybody else was feeling, to show my love, share the experience and help to support my family.

I would not have been able to do any of this had I been poorly, nor could I have hidden how I was feeling, as people who are very close to me can always see that I'm not well, even when I'm smiling and pretending everything is fine. Mum, especially, could see it in my eyes; she could even tell by my voice when I phoned her up. It would have made me feel very guilty if she'd had to worry about me on top of everything else, during such a difficult time.

I try not to dwell on it, but I sometimes wonder if my illness was responsible for my mum's cancer in the first place. I could see the pain that it caused her when my depression came on. I was so, so poorly and the effect on her was almost tangible.

She was diagnosed with the cancer two years after I became ill – and it's so often said that cancer is caused by stress. But when I asked the doctor who was treating her for his opinion, he said, 'No, let's be clear. Cigarettes caused your mother's cancer.'

Several years later, I was in a morning meeting at *Loose Women*, discussing what we would be talking about on the upcoming show. I wasn't feeling very well at the time and the topic of depression came up.

The actress and sometime *Loose Women* panellist, Terri Dwyer, was also in the meeting. Terri was having a really tough time, because her dad was very sick. 'What's to say that your depression is any worse than my depression?' she asked me.

'That's a really important question. Can we talk about it on the show rather than here?' I asked, because when we do a live show, I prefer everything I say to be spontaneous.

When we went on air, we explained that Terri's dad was dying of terminal illness, whereas nothing at all traumatic was happening in my life. 'I'm not saying that my depressive illness is worse than your sadness,' I said to Terri. 'I'm saying it's an illness, as opposed to yours, which isn't.

'If you went home tonight to find a doctor there, who told you, "We've found a cure for your dad. We're going to give him an injection and from tomorrow he'll get well," would your depression lift?'

'Well, of course it would,' she replied.

'Mine wouldn't,' I said. 'The difference is that if I was in a clinical depression and my dad happened to be ill, my depression would be the same whether he got better or he died. My depression is an inability to feel anything. It is not dependent on what is happening circumstantially.'

As I said this, I thought of my mum and how grateful I was that I hadn't become poorly while she was being treated for cancer. It gave me strength in years to come to remember that I could get through tough times emotionally without necessarily suffering depression.

IV

Grey, rainy, overcast weather has affected me for as long as I can remember. My friends at drama school used to call me a 'weather whinger' because I was always complaining about it.

'Shut up, man! We live in England, for God's sake!' they'd groan.

Back then, the weather didn't actually affect my body chemistry, but after I had post-natal depression, everything changed. Although my illness was mostly endogenous, certain things could bring it on, or help to bring it on, and the weather was among the things that made it worse. It was almost like having Seasonal Affective Disorder (SAD), without it being seasonal, of course, as our weather in the UK can be depressing all year round!

After the visitor made his first call, I developed an intense fear of grey, overcast days. As I watched the weather forecast, if I saw a black-grey cloud symbol over where I lived on the map my hands would start to tingle. I'd get the tinny taste in my mouth and pins and needles: all the signs of anxiety would kick in the moment I caught sight of that cloud.

Other people would just grumble, 'This bloody weather!', whereas I could feel my body chemistry changing and a greyness setting in.

I remember having some bad reactions to the weather while I was working on the ITV series, *Soldier Soldier*, which was a pity, because I enjoyed almost everything else about appearing in the show. *Soldier Soldier* was an award-winning drama about a group of soldiers in a fictional British Army regiment and was already hugely successful when I was cast in the role of Marsha Stubbs, in the third series. Marsha was the wife of the Command Sergeant Major, played by Rob Spendlove, and had some cracking storylines tied in with the other girls' shenanigans. The show was originally going to be called *Army Wives* and the female parts were really well written, which made it a delight. It was definitely a career breakthrough for me.

There were some fabulous people in the cast and we had a lot of fun filming on location in Germany and Cyprus. It was a special time because we knew we were creating something that people loved. It was also a sexy show; everybody who worked on it said so, and none of the actors who came over from the UK to make guest appearances ever wanted to leave!

ITV looked after us really well and in those days that meant looking after our families, too. If you were filming on location and had five days off or more, they would fly you home, or fly your family out. Tim and I were lucky that our work schedules usually allowed one or other of us to be at home with Matthew if the other was away, and the most I was ever apart from Matthew during the three years I was doing *Soldier Soldier* was a fortnight, once. On the rare occasions Tim and I were both away working, Matthew would stay with my sister or parents.

'My memories of my childhood are never that I felt lonely or that I missed you or Dad,' Matthew told me, a few years ago, 'because I was always around people who loved me.'

I missed being at home, but there was a lot to enjoy about being on location in the *Soldier Soldier* bubble. Many of us were drinkers, so it was like being sent on holiday with your best mates. I didn't feel at the time that I was drinking to self-medicate; I was doing it for social reasons, with my drinking gang, just to have fun. But inevitably I got poorly a few times, especially in Münster in Germany, where we filmed my first series and the sky was always cloudy and grey.

There was one particular day in Münster I remember waking up feeling very anxious. The weather was darkly overcast, the visitor was hovering and I just felt terrible. I looked at my schedule and saw that we were shooting a funeral scene later. It was one of those days when you knew there was not going to be much respite, just a lot of hanging around in a graveyard for hours on end.

First, though, we were filming in one of the houses on the army base. In the script, the scene was written as taking place on a sunny day, but it was so dark outside that the lighting guys had to use really strong halogen lights to create the illusion of bright daylight. When I went over to see how they were getting on, the glare and heat of the lights instantly warmed me. Having heard that halogen lights could help some people with depression, I closed my eyes and thought of sunny beaches in the hope that I would feel better, if only for a few moments. After that I did a lot of popping in to chat to the crew so that I could stand under the lights and wish myself off to the Caribbean. It didn't lift my depression, but I did it out of desperation.

Several years later I was given a SAD light, by the singer Chris de Burgh, of all people. He was a guest on *Down To Earth*, a series I did in 2004, and he was interested in hearing about my depression, especially as he had a friend who owned a halogen lighting company. Ever hopeful at first, I soon discovered that SAD lights don't actually help my depression in the way they help people with Seasonal Affective Disorder. Grrr! However, if I am feeling low and the weather is grey and horrible, sometimes I will go and have a sunbed and top up my Vitamin D – and maybe for the ten minutes I'm in there, I might feel a little better.

Mostly I didn't tell anyone when I was feeling ill, and nobody would have known, because I was good at pretending. But there was one awful time during my first series of *Soldier Soldier* when I couldn't hide it. We had two days off and a few of us made a plan to go off and stay at a chateau we'd discovered in the countryside. Since we were only allowed to travel within a certain radius of the set unless we had five days off, and this chateau was beyond our boundary, it felt a little bit naughty and exciting to be breaking the rules.

Hoping we wouldn't get caught, we didn't tell anybody where we were going. It was long before the days of, 'If you didn't Instagram it, it didn't happen.' You could keep secrets in a way that you can't now; life was so much easier then if you wanted to do something clandestine. I don't know how anybody does it any more – at least, anybody who's got a remotely recognisable face – because someone is bound to see them. I can't imagine getting away with anything: I only have to stop to get petrol and within a minute I'll see something on Twitter saying, 'Just seen Denise Welch at the Shell garage with her husband!'

I was really looking forward to our two days at the chateau – we all were. I got into the car: a normal, excited person, going on a sneaky trip. 'Can I stop and post a letter on the way?' I asked.

One of the gang said they knew of a post office just outside Münster, and so off we went.

Fifteen minutes into the journey, I thought, 'Wouldn't it be awful if the visitor came now?'

Horrified that I might have summoned him to me, I started moving around in an attempt to shake off the feeling that I might be getting poorly.

'Are you all right?' one of my friends asked.

'Yes, fine,' I said, my legs twitching.

Inside my head, my thoughts were going round like a tumble dryer: 'Yes, yes, yes, yes, yes, yes, I'm fine. I need to get out the car. I need to get out of the car. I need to get out the car.'

It was like mentally banging my head against a wall, or using a metaphorical TENS machine to distract me from the fear that I would get ill.

We pulled up in front of the post office, by which time the visitor was saying, 'I'm on my way to stop you having a nice time this weekend.'

'I'm going in the post office. I'm going in the post office. I'm going in the post office,' I chanted silently to myself.

I went inside the building and posted my letter. When I came out, I was almost catatonic. That's how quickly my depression can come on. I went from being a bright, bubbly, excited company member to being silent and withdrawn.

'What's wrong, Den?' my pals asked.

'It's my thing,' I said.

They knew about my illness, but of course it's one thing to know about it and another to see it go from nought to sixty in the time it took to post a letter.

'Shall we go back?' they said.

I shook my head. Although they didn't understand my illness and had never seen it before, they were people who cared about me and I felt I could be poorly in front of them. Also, being a people-pleaser, I was not going to be the one to let them down after all the excitement of the build-up to the weekend.

So we continued on the journey, and I kept asking them to stop the car so I could get out and vomit, in the hope that the physical act of being sick would take away the pain in my head. It gave me respite, however momentary, from how I was feeling. It was a trick I tried several times again in years to come.

When we arrived at the chateau, the depression lifted a little and went from grey-black to grey, so at least I could function and give the impression that I was okay for the next two days. But it was exhausting. People have no idea how physically gruelling an episode of depression is. Internally, you're fighting to survive against an opponent as strong as Tyson Fury. It depletes you of all your energy.

People who aren't ill often say to me, 'You've got to exercise more! It'll make you feel better.'

They don't realise that, when I'm coming out of a depression, I feel as if I've just climbed Everest. I'm so worn out from fighting it that I could fall asleep standing up. Consequently, there have been times in life when I can feel the visitor approaching and I don't have the energy to stop him. Instead I feel I have to give in.

'Right, you fucker, okay, do your worst!' I tell him. 'I can't fight you any more. I give up trying to shut the door in your face. In fact, I'm going to open it for you. There you go, come in. Ruin my life and fuck off.'

As long as he leaves, I know I'll be okay. Every time I am presented with a massive challenge with mental illness and I push through it, I build up strength for the next time.

'You were determined to bring me down,' I yell at him afterwards, 'and I still managed to go on, and I still managed to win awards, and I still managed to get good reviews, despite you. You were there all the time, but I still got through and achieved all of these things. So come on, I dare you: come at me again!'

If I can get through his visits, I can get through anything.

My storylines in *Soldier Soldier* were great when Marsha's husband Michael was a squaddie, but once he was promoted to officer and joined the posh ranks, in the fourth series, I suddenly found myself in the role of supportive wife making sandwiches in the kitchen. All I ever seemed to say was, 'Are you all right, darling? Would you like a tuna sandwich?'

I asked the producer to give my character something more interesting to do. Subsequently, Marsha hit a rocky patch in her marriage and became a club singer with a drink problem, which was much better than making sandwiches. I sang a Burt Bacharach number every week while stumbling around a nightclub, so it was a little bit like art mirroring life at times.

Some of the other characters decided to hold a talent show, and Marsha took part, which is how I came to sing the Dusty Springfield song, 'You Don't Have To Say You Love Me' on national television. They were only going to show a tiny clip of the song, but ultimately showed the whole thing.

Robson Green and Jerome Flynn were a bestselling pop duo by then. After singing 'Unchained Melody' on *Soldier Soldier*, they had been signed up by Simon Cowell, who at the time wasn't Simon Cowell, the famous *X Factor* person, but Simon Cowell, the head of the record company BMG. 'Unchained Melody' was a huge hit for BMG and there was a big buzz about the imminent Robson and Jerome debut album. Now word went round that I was going to be doing a turn in the upcoming fourth series of *Soldier Soldier*, and before I knew it, my agent had a call from Simon Cowell wanting to discuss releasing 'You Don't Have To Say You Love Me' as a single.

'You're not going to say yes?' my agent at the time asked, aghast.

She thought it was a totally naff idea and we nearly fell out over it. Not that having a pop career had ever been on the agenda for me, but if it was being offered to me on a plate, I was definitely going to think twice about turning it down.

'When is anyone ever again going to knock on the door to someone in her late thirties, who's not a singer, and say, "Do you want to make a record?"' I asked her. 'It's just not going to happen, so I'm going to do it.'

'That's not the point,' she said.

'Yes, it is,' I insisted.

I didn't think I was Aretha Franklin; it was more about ticking a box, having fun and telling my future grandchildren that Nana had once released a single.

My agent's assistant and my mum came with me to meet Simon Cowell, who was lovely. 'We'll get you on this and that show to promote the single,' he said enthusiastically. 'It's going to be great.'

My agent's assistant had his tongue in his cheek throughout the meeting, but I went away thinking, 'Simon Cowell is going to sign me!'

Then everything went quiet and I heard nothing from Simon Cowell ever again, not a solitary word. I later heard a rumour that BMG feared upsetting Robson if they signed up another person from *Soldier Soldier*. Whatever the real reason, I was absolutely fuming that my pop career was over before it had begun!

A couple of weeks later, Virgin Records swooped in and offered me a one-single deal. Just like that, my pop dreams rose up from the ashes. Off I went to Abbey Road Studios with Mike Batt of Wombles fame and recorded 'You Don't Have To Say You Love Me', accompanied by the BBC Philharmonic Orchestra, no less. I was straight on the phone to my mum and dad to tell them all about it, and years later, when Matthew also did some recording at Abbey Road with the BBC Philharmonic, he heard all about it, too!

All the recording and publicity for the single had to be timed around the talent contest episode of *Soldier Soldier*, which was airing in November 1995. I think Virgin saw me as a potential one-trick pony and didn't want to invest much money in promotional material, so they only gave me a very small budget to make a video. We had one day to shoot it, in Newcastle.

Since I could not take myself seriously as a pop star, I decided that the only way to do the video was to see it as a bit of fun. So I gathered as many famous people from the north-east as I could possibly muster in one place at one time, and the resulting random selection included: Willie Thorne and Dennis Taylor, the snooker players; Peter Beardsley, Lee Sharpe and Steve Watson, all footballers; Tim Healy, my famous actor husband; and the late, lovely Denise Robertson. My sister and I invited all of our pals along, and it was going to be Matthew's first onscreen appearance since he was a baby and bawled his head off throughout a whole scene of *Spender*.

We were filming in a club in South Shields and everyone was excited. Since nobody was getting paid, I wanted to create an upbeat, positive, 'Come on, we're all mucking in together for no money' feeling on the set. I was producing, co-directing and starring in the video, so there was quite a lot of pressure on me. On top of everything else, I organised the food and catering, as I felt the least I could do was make sure that people had a good day. As the shoot approached, I started feeling overwhelmed, and no wonder.

In the circumstances, the last thing I needed on the morning of the shoot was a call from the unwelcome visitor, wearing his grey cloak. When you consider that with depression it's hard enough work getting out of bed and having a shower, being the organising force behind a video shoot was like swimming to France in a force 7 storm.

I felt I couldn't let anybody know. I didn't even tell my nearest and dearest – not Tim, my sister, my mum or my dad – because I didn't want to ruin the day for anybody. They were all having such a laugh, especially my friends who didn't work in the industry, who were absolutely loving the fact that they were involved in something exciting like a pop video. Normally, I would have taken pleasure in the fun they were having. Yes, it would have been a stressful day – but I would have made it an enjoyable day and loved it, all the same.

As I was getting into my black sequinned dress, in my dressing room – and when I say 'dressing room,' I mean some insalubrious backstage area – I crouched down on the floor and fervently prayed that the depression would lift. 'Yet again,' I thought, 'something that should be a wonderful memory, a fun memory, is marred by you being here.'

It just ruined it for me.

Luckily, my friends and family have great memories of the day, and when you look at the video, you would never know what was going on behind the scenes, not in a million years. All this time later, I'm proud to say that my single went to number 23 in the charts – and although the video didn't fare quite so well, it has since become a cult promo on the naff-videos circuit and I consider it a badge of honour that on YouTube it is included in a compilation of the 'Top 10 Worst Ever Pop Videos'! I'd rather be in the top 10 of something than nothing.

V

When I look back on how hard it has been to live with depression, I often think how difficult life would be as a single parent with this illness, or someone with no support, doing a relentless job: working in a fish factory, maybe, or tapping endlessly at a keyboard in a hi-tech computer environment.

It makes me realise how lucky I am to do a job I love, even though acting presents a lot of challenges to somebody who has a depressive illness. Unlike a lot of people, when I'm working I can't take a day off if I'm ill. Not because I won't get paid, but because as many as 200 people – cast and crew – will be depending on me. If I'm in a play and I don't turn up, unless there's an understudy the show can't go on; if I'm filming a scene for television, even an understudy wouldn't be able to take my place and do it for me.

My job is rarely boring, but it can be high-pressure, and in television there's nowhere tougher to work than a long-running TV soap opera. So although I was over the moon to be cast in *Coronation Street*, my next big job after *Soldier Soldier* – and it went on to be a fantastic job for me and a fabulous few years, all told – I found the reality of filming four episodes a week quite gruelling, and sometimes overwhelming. The schedule was unstoppable, and even more so by the time I left, when we were filming five episodes a week. Bearing in mind that film actors usually have a couple of months to make a movie, working on a soap is the equivalent of making two full-length movies in a week. You get no rehearsal time: you're straight in there; quick run-through, record.

I was warned at my audition that the part of Natalie Horrocks had a shelf life, but I didn't care: I was such a huge fan of *Coronation Street* that I would have been happy just to do a couple of scenes if it meant I could say I'd been in *Corrie*. I could hardly believe that I would be working alongside people I had admired all my life: actors like Bill Roache (Ken Barlow), Liz Dawn (Vera Duckworth) and Barbara Knox (Rita Fairclough). Legends, all!

Soap operas have their ebbs and flows and *Coronation Street* needed a bit of a boost when Natalie turned up and started having an affair with (married) Kevin Webster, one of the street's stalwarts, played by Michael Le Vell. Natalie was only supposed to be around for seventeen episodes, but she soon became a character that viewers loved to hate. People were mesmerised by the way she lured Kevin into her web; audience figures rose and, before I knew it, my contract had been extended by three months.

I was the first person to go into *Coronation Street* with an established public profile, having already appeared in *Spender* and *Soldier Soldier*. So I had experienced fame up to a point – 'Oh my God, you're in *Soldier Soldier*! Can I have your autograph?'

Since 20 million people were watching *Corrie*, however (and 25 million for the fortieth-anniversary live episode), I suddenly found myself at another level of fame altogether. Everybody in the country seemed to know who I was. People would nearly faint when they saw me. They would scream in my face. I couldn't walk down the street.

At the same time, life was pretty lonely. After the fun and frolics of being part of the *Soldier Soldier* drinking gang, I couldn't get used to the way most of the *Corrie* cast members ducked off home at the end of the day. I could understand it, as most of them lived in the Manchester area, so their homes and families were nearby, but it didn't make it any easier for me, living in a rented flat in Castleford, a long way from Matthew and Tim in Northumberland. I am blessed with a wonderful family and circle of friends, and I missed the warmth and activity of my social life at home. One night, I was so desperate for company that I sat in the bar of the Victoria & Albert Hotel in Manchester, nursing a drink, reading a newspaper and pretending to be waiting for a friend. I was hoping that someone I knew would come in: I could say I'd been let down by a pal, and have a drink with them instead. But nobody came.

Later on, I had some great times and made some fantastic friends at *Coronation Street*, but I can't deny that I struggled with my mental health for much of the time I worked there. This wasn't because of the relentless workload, which was incredibly busy and involved juggling lots of balls, for me and many of the other actors. If it became overwhelming at times, it was because of my illness; I didn't blame *Coronation Street*, because it was clear to me that I had no control of when it came. Still, my first six months there were really tough and in the years to come there were times when I honestly didn't know if I was going to make it through.

Alcohol definitely made things worse, although at the time I didn't realise how much worse. I drank a lot, reaching for anything that I thought would take away the pain of my illness and keep me going through the long days. It was very different from the fun, social drinking of my time on *Soldier Soldier*. This was drinking to self-medicate my illness and lift my feelings of isolation and loneliness.

Drinking for fun is a world away from drinking with depression. When you're going out with your girlfriends and you're sharing a bottle of fizzy as you're getting ready – having a laugh, feeling tipsy and dancing around the bedroom – that's alcohol at its best, enhancing the happy mood you're in. It engulfs your brain in endorphins and triggers a positive feeling in your body. You feel dizzy and excited; it's brilliant. Drinking with depression felt nothing like that. It was a horrible type of drinking, a deadening, a pain-killer; it was never to do with feeling tipsy or having fun. When you're depressed, you long to feel normal and alcohol makes you feel closer to normal. It didn't make the depression go away; it just put me into kind of a dead zone and made an evening out more bearable.

While you're drinking, your brain adapts to the changes that alcohol causes, but when you stop, it reacts the other way, leading to a dip in endorphins – if you're normal – and a terrifying plummet to the depths of depression if you're dealing with an existing imbalance in brain chemistry. This plummet caused my terrible hangovers and, despite the fact that I couldn't shake them off like everybody else – with a fatty fry-up breakfast and ten gallons of tea – I could not resist the temptation to drink again in the evening and make the pain go away. I still wasn't a daytime drinker, but I'd make up for it after work.

During the day I often hid away in my dressing room, wishing the day away, sleeping or pretending I was asleep, staying out of sight so that I didn't have to talk to anyone, only coming out of my room when I needed to. I didn't want people to see how poorly I was. They'd only blame it on my nights of partying.

So, although people say that you shouldn't have regrets, I think it's impossible not to. When I look back to that time, I think, 'Why didn't I realise that alcohol was making my depression a lot worse? Why didn't I just stop drinking?'

I know why, of course. For the two or three hours that I was actually consuming alcohol, it obliterated my illness. That is why so many people with depression drink. People who drink normally, who don't have a problem with alcohol, walk through the door after a stressful day, saying, 'Oh my God, just get me a glass of wine!' It takes the edge off – and that's what it did for me, except that I always needed more; I didn't have an off-button. Whereas normal people think, 'I've had a great night and now it's time to go to bed,' the depressive and the alcoholic go on chasing the feeling alcohol gives them, and often that's simply the desire to *not feel pain*.

For me, my issues with drinking started with self-medication and grew into alcoholism – or was it the other way round? It's the chicken or the egg, again: alcohol causes depression. Depression causes alcoholism – and I was fast becoming an alcoholic.

Natalie, my character, lived off the set and her scenes at home had to be filmed at a real house in Chorlton on a Sunday. This meant that I often had to come back down to Manchester from Northumberland on a Saturday night, having only driven home on the Friday night. It broke my heart to say goodbye to Matthew and get in the car. 'Is it worth it?' I asked myself, every time, tears streaming down my face. 'But of course it's worth it,' I'd tell myself. 'I'm in the greatest, longest-running soap opera of all time!'

I was thrilled when my *Corrie* contract was extended by a year, but felt I couldn't bear being apart from Tim and Matthew any longer. After getting an unofficial nod from my boss that Natalie was likely to be in the show for the long haul, I persuaded Tim to move down from Northumberland to Wilmslow in Cheshire, where my mum's sister, my Auntie Julie, was living. Tim wasn't happy about it, but he came, albeit kicking and screaming, and we settled in Wilmslow, a town that Tim complained was 'so posh, it's got its own bloody credit card!'

Things were much better after we rented a house opposite where Auntie Julie and my cousins lived, although I didn't see much of it or them, because you pretty much live on set when you're a regular character in a TV soap. You're usually up around five in the morning, at the studios for make-up at seven and on set at eight. I was getting up in darkness at the crack of dawn, going straight in to work and getting home fourteen hours later, only just in time to put Matthew to bed. That was my life, most of the time. People said, 'It must be lovely having Matty on the doorstep now,' but on weekdays I barely saw him.

Matthew's new school was putting a lot of pressure on him as well, bless his little heart. I'd come home from work, absolutely shattered, and he'd be poring over some incredibly hard maths homework. I desperately wanted to be there for my child and spend time with him, but too often we ended up doing this awful, frustrating homework together, made all the worse by the fact that I haven't been able to do maths since I left Reception!

All things considered, my first year at *Coronation Street* was a very challenging time and it's no surprise to me that I suffered from crushing depression and had what I consider to be a full mental breakdown. It seemed very unfair. I was in my dream job but felt too poorly to relish it, and a lot of landmark days were ruined. I'll never forget when Natalie started working at the Rovers Return, just after I'd signed a contract to stay in the show for a further year. The night before my debut as a barmaid, my dad phoned me and said, 'It's so exciting, isn't it? We can't wait to see you behind the bar of the Rovers!'

'Yes, it's great,' I said, feeling nothing but flat depression.

The next evening, I watched the episode alone with the unwelcome visitor, seething with resentment. 'You've ruined another massive milestone in my life, you bastard,' I told him. 'I'm the barmaid of the Rovers Return in *Coronation Street* – and I feel nothing.'

After spending several really bad days with the visitor, I would have expected him to leave. This time, however, he hung around longer than usual, because something monumental happened – something that affected me so badly that he had an excuse to stay.

Early on Sunday morning, 31 August 1997, my cousin Steve came over to borrow a stepladder. I answered the door in a daze of depression.

'God, it's bloody awful about Diana, isn't it?' he said.

'What?' I asked.

'Princess Diana has died. Didn't you hear it on the radio?'

This knocked me sideways. Like millions of people on that sunny Sunday morning, I just could not believe that such tragic news could be true. I was already having a weird time with my illness; now everything became ten times weirder. It felt as if the world had changed – and I had a dread of things changing whenever I was poorly. I went back into the house and called my sister, who told me that Dodi Fayed had died alongside Diana. It was just awful.

I rang work and said, 'You can't make us work today.'

But of course we did have to go to work.

I was filming in 'Firman's Freezers', with Kevin Webster's character, played by Michael Le Vell, all day, which was totally surreal. This huge public figure had died and everybody was getting on with normal life. I'm not saying that Michael Le Vell didn't care about Diana dying – I'm sure he did – but I remember seeing him having a laugh about something later in the day and it just seemed so strange to me. If I'd been a character in a film at that moment, the camera would have pulled back to show me watching a montage of people laughing and being completely normal, while I was trapped inside a bubble of depression in a world that had changed for ever.

The following day, a load of us were booked to go to London for the *TV Quick* Awards, where Sally Whittaker and I were presenting an award. 'You're not seriously going to make us go, are you?' I asked Brian, one of the producers, who was also a good friend.

He shrugged his shoulders. Life goes on, and so do awards ceremonies. We had no choice but to attend.

There was a deathly hush throughout the whole country during the week after Diana died. Even people who weren't depressed must have found it strange dealing with the horrible, surreal atmosphere, while for me, and no doubt for others like me, that weird feeling coupled with clinical depression was off the scale. I don't know how I got through the awards night without running away, although it was probably because I didn't know where to run. When I'm depressed and away from home, I have to be able to visualise getting back to my safe places, to my bed or my sofa – but now it felt as if there was nowhere safe to go.

The next two weeks were very difficult. Although I had met several members of the Royal Family I had never met Princess Diana, and yet her death felt like a personal bereavement, as it did for millions of other people. I still to this day don't know why.

I watched the funeral on television at home. For me, the worst moment was seeing the coffin and the flowers saying, 'Mummy'. That word made me collapse onto the kitchen floor and start wailing with grief. Even though, like a lot of women, I related to Diana in many ways, it seems like a complete overreaction to the death of someone I didn't know. I think it was a manifestation of my illness, on top of not being able to process what was happening, but it was awful: I couldn't understand where these loud, heart-wrenching sobs were coming from.

Then everything went red. It was as if someone had painted a hazy red filter over my eyes. The floor was red, the walls were red: even the trees outside the kitchen window were red. 'Agh, I'm going mad!' I screamed, pushing myself along the floor into one corner of the kitchen, where I curled up into a ball.

I was terrified. It felt like proper madness.

My heart was pounding. I was in a state of utter panic. Suddenly, the words of my wonderful mother popped into my head. 'People who go mad don't know they're going mad,' she used to say. 'As long as you're saying, "I'm going mad", you're not going mad.'

As I blinked red, and then red again, I clung to Mum's words for comfort. If you think you're going mad, you're not going mad.

Never forget it.

This was the first of several mental breakdowns to come. These were caused by my illness and my desperate attempts to self-medicate in the absence of having time off to de-compress.

A couple of days later, somebody offered me some cocaine. 'You are in a terrible state,' they said. 'This will make you feel better.'

As anybody with severe clinical depression will know, in that position you will do anything to stop the pain. This was behind my first use of cocaine and, unfortunately for me, it seemed to work better than alcohol at relieving my depression.

It was, however, very temporary. A line of cocaine gave me forty minutes of feeling normal. Then, scared of coming down, I'd have another.

Each line of cocaine made for a worse eventual comedown. I sometimes stayed awake through the night and into the morning, because I was so terrified of the crash. I'd go into work without having had a wink of sleep and, as the morning progressed, a horrendous hangover would set in, making me feel much more poorly than before. All the while I did my best to hide what was happening to me from my colleagues and bosses, while trying – and succeeding – to be consistently

good at my job. It amazes me how I managed to be a successful actress while all of this was going on.

As a rule, I don't look back and dwell on the bad days of my
depression: I try to focus on the times in between. Yet there
are certain milestones I can't forget, my fortieth birthday cele-
bration being among them.

It was 1998 and I was having a big party, which was being
covered by a magazine; this was the sort of thing you were
encouraged to do in those days if you were in a famous TV
soap. It was back when the magazines would give you quite
good money in exchange for coverage – as long as you got a
few celebrities along – which meant you could throw a more
lavish party than you would have done otherwise.

A few days before the party, I started getting stressed. This
wasn't because I was thinking, 'Oh my God, there's a lot of
work to do with this party,' it was, 'Oh my God, wouldn't it be
awful if I got ill?'

I couldn't help it. It took many years to develop a strategy
to stop myself panicking in this way – and I was still a long
way off finding it. 'Why do I put myself in these situations?' I
asked myself angrily.

Nobody was forcing me to have a fortieth birthday party; I
was doing it voluntarily. But why, when I knew the fear of the
fear could ruin everything? It was almost as if I'd set myself
up for a fall.

The party was being held at a beautiful spa hotel in
Cheshire called Mottram Hall and I'd invited people from
my present life and my past life. My friendship groups
haven't really changed very much over the years and the
guest list included lots of different sets of friends, including
my oldest and best mates from the north-east. So, as well as
being my fortieth, it was also going to be a reunion of all my
old school pals.

I remember Rob, one of my ex-boyfriends from my school-days, calling up and saying, 'We can't wait for Saturday! We've been talking about it for weeks.'

He wasn't to know it, but saying something like that would start an anxiety in me, because I felt a pressure to be well on the day. 'All these people are really looking forward to it!' I thought. 'I mustn't get ill.'

At work, people were saying, 'You all sorted for Saturday, Den? What are you wearing?'

These were normal questions about normal things, but they made me panic inside. Before long, I could sense the unwelcome visitor making his way to my side.

The night before my party, I had a drink in the hope that I might be able to calm my fears about being poorly. In my panic I drank too much, and the next morning I woke up to that lethal combination: a hangover and depression.

I dressed, got in the car and drove to Carrs, a big local park, planning to make the pain stop by running off both the hangover and my depression.

I'm not a great runner – in fact, I'm a terrible runner – but I ran for my life that day. I ran like hell, as if the visitor was chasing me, pushing myself faster and further in a desperate attempt to throw him off and leave him behind.

It didn't work.

In the films, when people don't want to go ahead with the party, they just get in their cars and drive off. Unfortunately, that doesn't happen in real life! I probably had 200 people arriving at Mottram Hall Hotel for my party. I wanted to run away like never before, but I had to go through with it; I had no choice.

It was dreadful, literally – I was filled with dread, knowing that people would be expecting and wanting me to be on sparkling form that night, because that's the person the non-depressed me would be. Meanwhile, I just wanted to withdraw. The thought of doing anything with depression is just so hard.

I spent the evening pretending to be sparkling Denise. I drank all night and just about got through it. To everyone else, it was a fantastic party, but my memory of it is horrific and the next day I felt absolutely awful. I had people staying at my house and when I woke up in the morning, they were making breakfast and roaring with laughter at every hilarious moment they could recall as they dissected the evening. Once again, my illness had sucked all the fun out of a special day.

Shortly after this, we moved out of our big rented house into Rose Cottage, which became our family house for the next decade. I loved Rose Cottage and have many happy memories of living there, but there were dark times too. I had my second serious breakdown not long after we moved in. My illness was so bad that I would wake up in the morning, after very little sleep, in a thick, black depression, and I would crawl to the toilet on my hands and knees, shaking and sweating and unable to think, knowing that I had to go to work. Then, even though I didn't feel sick, I would put my fingers down my throat and make myself vomit, hoping that the ten seconds of relief I got from it would take away some of what was going on in my head.

Those horrendous mornings gave me an understanding of why people self-harm: for the displacement, to take the pain away from your head by causing pain somewhere else. For me, the next step could easily have been something like cutting. I never did it – thank God – but I understand the origin of the feeling that drives people to it.

By now, I was one of the most regular *Coronation Street* cast members: Natalie had become the landlady of the Rovers and I was always behind the bar. It was very rare that I had a day off, or even a morning, and I didn't consider taking time off for mental illness. I should have been kinder to myself, but when you're working in a TV show, you can't ring in sick and Sue on the other computer will do your job for the day. The show comes to a halt without you. There's no escaping it.

I drank heavily to self-medicate through the breakdown, so my life was one long vicious circle: I was on a wheel that I couldn't get off: depression, self-medication, hangover, depression. Nobody had much sympathy for me, because they saw me drinking and assumed that my problems were self-inflicted. There was still a lot of ignorance and misunderstanding around mental illness then and I felt isolated – or just apart – for much of the time. It is tough when you can't tell people at work how you're feeling.

This is still a big problem today. Although things are getting better, talking about depression in the workplace is not easy for many people, because of the widespread misconceptions about what depression actually is.

PART 3

Self-medicating

I

I didn't go from being a little wallflower to being an outrageous, self-medicating drinker overnight. Being a party
animal is in my DNA; I had party animal parents and I took
after them.

My parents, Annie and Vin, were twenty-one when I was
born and the upside of this was that my sister, Debbie, and I
never missed out on their company, because they used to take
us everywhere with them. Mum and Dad loved having fun
and lived life to the full. They had lots of friends and were
social drinkers: they got drunk at parties, but they didn't sit
around drinking in front of the television.

They were forever having their friends over on Friday and
Saturday nights. I have a strong memory of standing in the
doorway of the lounge at our house in Monkseaton, just
outside Whitley Bay, asking plaintively, 'When is everybody
going to go home?'

In my mind it was four o'clock in the morning, but it was
probably only about eleven at night! I've equated the night-
time with drama and excitement ever since those days.

One evening, aged six, I appeared on the stairs at home and
said, 'Come on, let's all go to the Rex!'

The Rex was a posh hotel on the promenade in Whitley
Bay, where Mum and Dad had their first date. It held a huge
allure for me.

Mum said I could never understand why she sent me to
bed when her friends came over. What on earth would they be

doing or saying that I couldn't share in? And surely my presence could only enhance their evening? I used to come downstairs and try to join in with the girls' talk, telling jokes, reciting poems and taking sips from people's wine glasses when I thought they weren't looking.

I must have picked this up from Dad, who has the worst FOMO of anyone I've known. He still has it, and it drives me up the bloody wall. It's stressful, because my children don't want me to have anything to do with their social lives any more, but I have a father who expects me to have a teenage-style plan of campaign for his nights out.

Dad still looks at me as if to say, 'What, we're going home now, and it's only one o'clock in the morning?' He was gutted recently when he missed a wedding after-party in someone's hotel room at four in the morning. 'I wish I hadn't gone to bed at two!' he complained bitterly at breakfast the following morning.

'Dad, you're eighty-three!' I said.

Mum was very stylish, and very funny, and her creativity came out in the way she dressed. She was always glamorous, always fashionably ahead of her time. I took after her in that when I grew up, I loved a drink and a fag. My sister didn't get that gene – she feels sick and her head starts spinning after two glasses of wine.

Dad is and always has been an entertainer and exhibition-ist. He is the life and soul of the party, and I never questioned the fact that he liked to dress up as a woman and burst into song, given half the chance. He used to do a bit of a drag act as Raquel (as in Raquel Welch, although that reference seems to completely go over people's heads now), and my sister and I were also used to seeing him come downstairs as Shirley Bassey. Debbie was always horrified by this, in a tongue-in-cheek way. I, however, used to think it was very normal, as normal as it was to have Ian La Frenais pull up at our front door in a Silver Cloud Rolls-Royce. Rather randomly, before he wrote *The Likely Lads*, *Porridge* and *Auf Wiedersehen, Pet*, Ian La Frenais was Uncle Ian, my godfather, living at the end of the road with his parents, Auntie Gladys and Uncle Cyril. Later on, I was rather dazzled by him. When *The Likely Lads* was being filmed, one of the stars of the series, Rodney Bewes, was staying with us, and Ian, Rodney and Tom Courtenay picked me up from my junior school in the Silver Cloud and took me for fish and chips in Whitley Bay. When I got out of the car to go back to school, I said, 'Ah well, back to reality!', a line Rodney Bewes quoted many years later when he came on my *This Is Your Life*.

Debbie and I grew up surrounded by creativity and people who always seemed to be having a great time. Parties and socialising were part of that and I equated drinking with having fun. It was only after post-natal depression opened me up to the pain of depression that I started using alcohol to self-medicate my mental pain.

'When you talk about your drinking days, it's always related to pain, heartbreak and depression,' one of my friends said to me recently. 'You must cut yourself some slack and remember that we also had some good times.'

She's right. I think of alcohol as being the devil, and yet there were some great times. I think the nights when I was able to leave it at just being a bit tipsy were probably fine, but as time went on I couldn't really drink socially. Even if I knew I had work the next day, I couldn't stop. It was a classic case of, 'One wasn't enough, two was too many.'

'Well, that's me, then,' were words I never said. Someone clearly forgot to programme them into my computer at birth.

When I was asked to appear on a celebrity special of *Stars in Their Eyes* in 1999, I wasn't sure at first if *Coronation Street* would let me do it, as some soap operas can be quite fussy about what their cast members get up to; but I was lucky and my bosses were quite lenient with me. Not only did they agree to me doing *Stars in Their Eyes,* but the following year they also gave me permission to present a DIY series, as baffling as that may sound. To this day it makes me chuckle to think that, at one point in the history of television, a group of people from a TV production company, after learning that they'd got the commission to make a series called *The Real DIY Show,* were sitting round a table and somebody said, 'I know, let's ask Denise Welch, that famous DIY expert!'

When *The Real DIY Show with Denise Welch* was launched, there were posters all over town showing a photo of me holding a drill, next to the strapline, 'Licensed to drill!' Now, whenever I see a TV star or personality incongruously linked with a show, I wonder, 'How did they decide on that particular person? How on earth did that person get the job?'

Taking part in a singing competition was nowhere near as big a stretch since, although I've never considered myself a singer or a musical theatre artist, I've often described myself as an actress who can hold a tune. However, having now appeared in several musicals, including the West End production of *Yakety Yak,* a stint as Sandy in *Grease* and a nationwide tour of *Calendar Girls: The Musical,* I'm more confident in my singing ability and should perhaps be less self-deprecating about my abilities.

The regular, non-celebrity *Stars in Their Eyes* series had been running successfully for nearly a decade and featured contestants impersonating famous singers. The format never varied: first you saw a contestant being interviewed as they really were; then they said, 'Tonight, Matthew, I'm going to be . . .' The next shot was of them emerging through a cloud of dry ice, totally transformed into a pop or cabaret star. Glenda Wood, the head of make-up at Granada TV, wrought some truly incredible transformations, and there was a lot of fun to be had in judging how much someone looked or sounded like the performer they were imitating.

After I was given the go-ahead to appear on the show, it was decided that I would be Petula Clark and sing 'Downtown'. I wish I'd done someone different, though, because my hair was already short and blonde, so when I came through the clouds I simply looked like me with a different dress on. You didn't see the huge transformation that you saw with some people.

I enjoyed the rehearsals, which were held across the road from *Coronation Street* and fitted in easily with my downtime. It was fun having time out of my day job to do something different. I had a singing coach, who was fabulous to work with, and although I was nervous in the months leading up to the show, I drew comfort from the thought that there had previously been several celebrity *Stars in Their Eyes* contestants who weren't brilliant singers. So it was all quite exciting, especially as my entire family were coming down for the studio day.

The week before the show, I started feeling very anxious and could hardly eat. People assumed it was performance nerves and kept saying, 'It'll be fine. You can sing. I've seen you in rehearsals. You're doing a great job.'

They were very well-meaning, but it wasn't about that. I was nervous, yes, but more than anything I was worried that the visitor would arrive and jeopardise my performance. 'Don't you dare come and ruin things for me on this TV show,' I warned him, over and over again.

The night before the big day, I was staying at the V&A Hotel, a hotel that was synonymous with Manchester, *Coronation Street* and wild parties. Dear God, the times that I woke up in the bar of the V&A Hotel, surrounded by drunken pals! Things had changed a lot in the two years since I had sat there alone all evening, hoping to bump into somebody I knew.

On this particular night, the other *Stars in Their Eyes* contestants were also staying at the V&A because we had a very early start in the morning for camera rehearsals. Harry Hill, who was impersonating Morrissey, Kirsty Young (Peggy Lee), Ben Freeman (Robbie Williams) and Michelle Collins (Chrissy Hynde) were all there. Meanwhile, I could feel the visitor coming and knew there was nothing I could do about it.

These days I do everything I can to lessen my illness. I've made changes in my life, including stopping drinking, that have helped me manage it a lot better. Yet I will always understand why people self-medicate, because although I knew from experience that I would feel much worse the next day, my depression was often so bad that all I could think about was stopping the pain, if only for a few short hours.

This is what happened that night at the V&A, when I bumped into an acquaintance who had been a guest artist on *Soldier Soldier* and had a drink with him.

Hindsight is, of course, a wonderful thing, but if that was me now, I wouldn't sit at the bar, thinking, 'I'm going to drink and obliterate everything.'

Instead, I'd say to myself, 'You feel terrible, Denise, but don't drink and compound it, because you might just be able to arrest this. You might just be able to stop the visitor coming if you go to bed now.'

Back then, I didn't have the tools to think clearly and act in my own best interest. I was beyond anxious and so I went for the easy route, which was to have a drink. It's not an excuse, but it was how I used to try to quell what was happening to me. One drink led to another and, since I had no off-button, I very foolishly got hammered. It was the most unprofessional thing I could have done.

When I woke up in the morning, I felt so horrendous that I wanted to jump out of the window of the hotel. I was hungover and my depression was at full pelt, because the drinking had accelerated it – that's what alcohol always did. Although I would have undoubtedly had depression on the day of the show anyway, do I think I would have had it as badly as I did without alcohol? No, absolutely not, because there was also a self-hating, self-destructive aspect to getting drunk in that situation.

Any normal person would have woken up on the morning of the show and thought, 'What a stupid cow. Why did I have those drinks? I feel like shit,' but by midday, after a bag of chips, they would have felt fine again.

Whereas I was at an all-time, desperate low. Ahead of me lay a day and night that should have been exciting and fun, albeit really stressful, but would now be shrouded in depression. I faced long, long hours of pretending everything was fine. 'Why have I done this to myself?' I asked myself despairingly. 'It's just made it worse. I can't remember anything!'

I made it to the studios and into the dressing room. As I went through the motions of putting on my blue, Petula Clark minidress, several people said, 'Wow, you look amazing. Your legs are so thin! You've lost weight for this, haven't you, to look like her?'

'Yes, yes,' I said, shying away from the subject. In fact, my weight was low because my periods of depression had been so bad that I couldn't eat anything.

I've always loved my food and have never been very controlled about what I eat. Therefore, in my periods of wellness, I would be queuing at the butty wagon, eating chips and pie at lunchtime: I wasn't a salad muncher; I was a salad dodger. But one of the first things to go when I'm in depression is my appetite. It has always, sadly, been a little bit of a silver lining – but I didn't revel in it, or think I looked amazing. I wasn't unhealthily thin – I was a size 8 – and yet I was aware that people were complimenting me simply because I was slim, not because I looked well. I can't have looked well.

On a typical production day, you're taken to make-up. You're taken to hair. You're taken to wardrobe. You're taken to do a camera rehearsal. So you're traipsing all over the building, and on this day, as I moved robotically from one place to the next, my depression was so thick that my mouth started to stiffen and I became incapable of talking properly.

'She's really nervous, this one! She normally never shuts up,' remarked Glenda in make-up, who was a real barrel of fun, but such a powerhouse that she could be quite scary too.

'Yes, I know,' I said, barely able to speak. 'I'm not feeling too . . .'

I wanted to explain that I wasn't feeling nervous in the normal way. The 'normal me' would have been standing backstage, buzzing with the usual performance nerves, saying to Kirsty Young and Harry Hill, 'What are we doing this for? Are we crazy?' while thinking, 'Oh my God, my heart is racing. Oh no, please, I don't want to go on!'

This was completely different. I was in such dark depression that when I got back to my dressing room, I started crawling around and banging my head on the floor, trying desperately to deaden the pain within. At one point, I got into the wardrobe and sat there, my head buried in my hands; I don't know why. The pain was excruciating. I was beside myself. I didn't know what else to do.

I was in this state when Matthew Kelly came to see me, Matthew being the beloved host of *Stars in Their Eyes*. Someone had told him that I was really nervous.

I knew Matthew from bumping into him at TV shows and industry events. In other words, I didn't know him very well. He sat down opposite me. 'What is the matter?' he asked. 'You're going to be fine, you know.'

'Matthew, it's not nerves. It's anxiety,' I said.

He didn't register the difference. He started reassuring me as if I was nervous about going on, which was kind of him, and I made the right noises to make him think he was calming me down. I didn't feel I could explain that my body chemistry had completely messed me up; nor did I want to admit that I'd gone out the night before and felt responsible for bringing on an episode of major depression by drinking too much.

'I'll be fine, I'll be fine, I'll be fine,' I told him, because I had to be fine.

There was no alternative. I couldn't back out now. Yet, standing in my dressing room after he'd gone, trying to sing 'Downtown', I still couldn't move my mouth properly.

Everything was taking longer that day because they had a problem with the jib, the camera that swings and swoops from left to right on a crane across the set. So the audience, who had come in expecting to be there for a couple of hours, ended up being there for six. My family; my friends Steven and Lester: everybody was there, waiting and waiting.

Engulfed in depression, I didn't want to see any of them before I went on, because it would have made me feel even worse than I already did. Fortunately I had the pretext that I didn't want to spoil the surprise by revealing my transformed state – even though, in fact, I didn't look any different.

The next few hours were like a nightmare version of something that should have been exciting. I did my interview with Matthew Kelly and said, 'And tonight, Matthew, I'm going to be Petula Clark.'

Then it was off into make-up for a couple of hours before I reappeared through the dry ice. While the lovely make-up girls bustled around being their bubbly, jubilant selves, I did my best to smile at them with my dead eyes.

Eventually, the time came to appear through the cloud of dry ice. Conscious that everybody who'd already gone before me had delivered a great performance, I stood on the stage, feeling as if I was in a parallel universe, as the voiceover said, 'And tonight, ladies and gentlemen, Petula Clark!'

I walked through the dry ice, the band began playing and I started singing 'Downtown', trying to remember the words and sing them in the style of Petula Clark. To my relief, I got through it. The audience duly clapped. Then I had to do a second take.

'You did brilliantly, considering you were so nervous,' someone said afterwards.

'Could you tell?' I asked.

While I was singing, apparently, my hand and my microphone were shaking so uncontrollably that it looked like I was giving someone a handjob! Normally I would have worked out a technique to control it, but I couldn't do anything about it in the state I was in.

Kirsty Young won as Peggy Lee. She was fabulous. What's funny is that her husband sent me a card afterwards, saying, 'Hi, Denise, it's Nick Jones, Kirsty's husband. I just wanted to thank you for being so lovely to Kirsty, because she was incredibly nervous.'

'Wow!' I thought, because I couldn't remember a thing about reassuring Kirsty.

'In all my years of doing *Celebrity Stars in Their Eyes*, I never saw anybody as nervous as Denise Welch,' Matthew Kelly wrote, years later.

It didn't really matter that he had misinterpreted what had happened. I was used to people not getting it. What annoyed me a tiny bit was that anybody reading his words would think that I was this crazy, nervous person, which I wasn't.

I was clinically depressed.

II

The trouble with writing a memoir about depression is that focusing on my illness makes it seem as if every event in my life over the last thirty years has been horrendous, and of course that is not the case! Life is full of joy and laughter when I'm not ill, and involves all the usual ups and downs. I'm not someone who sits around and dwells on what could have been; when I'm well, I'm out there making the most of life. A recent weekend in London springs to mind as I write this, when I took my sister and nieces to *Mamma Mia The Party* at the O2 on the Friday night, went with my dad to RuPaul's first ever UK DragCon all day on the Saturday and went to DragCon again on the Sunday with Matthew and his new girlfriend, when I introduced Baga Chipz. Prior to this, my dad had been treated to an all-expenses-paid VIP trip to Stringfellows on the Friday night. There was no stopping him if you'd wanted to! It was the most amazing weekend.

There have been lots of periods of wellness, and there have also been times when I've been convinced I would be ill, but wasn't. I didn't have one depressive episode while making *The Real DIY Show with Denise Welch*, for instance, or during the massive highs and lows I experienced while doing *Dancing On Ice* in 2011.

Still, there's no denying that a lot of special days were spoiled by the presence of my unwelcome visitor, and I'm writing about them here as a kind of reckoning. I'm putting them down in black and white in defiance of him, to show him that he hasn't beaten me and will never triumph over me, however hard he makes life for me. I want other people who suffer from depression to know that they can get through it – as I do and have done and will continue to do. I want to show them how bad it has been, but that I've survived.

Even as every call from the visitor darkened my world, I was gradually inching my way towards the light, moving closer to making the changes in my life that would diminish my chances of getting depression. These days, light has a much stronger presence in my life than darkness, but for years, self-medicating with alcohol often cast black shadows of its own.

Around the same time I did *Stars in Their Eyes*, I was due to go to London to open a car expo in Earl's Court, which was the sort of thing you did if you were in the number-one soap on television, watched by 20 million people.

Out of the blue, Tim announced, rather bizarrely, 'I'm going to come with you.'

'Why? I thought you had something else you were doing?' I said.

'No, no, I can do it another time. I want to come with you,' he insisted.

It wasn't that we never did anything together, but the opening of a car expo wasn't the sort of thing he would normally come to, and there was no need for him to be there, either, because everything had been organised in advance and I was going to be well looked after.

Later it transpired that my agent, Barry, had said to Tim, 'You must go with her, because we don't want her to drink.'

I didn't drink every day, but when I did drink I became powerless over it – and of course at these big events, people were constantly saying, 'Would you like a glass of champagne? Glass of champagne? Glass of champagne?'

I didn't have a cut-off point and I think Barry and Tim had visions of me phoning up from London, saying, 'I've met this great bunch of people and we're all going to Soho House and then we're going to a nightclub together, and then . . .'

As long as I knew that Matthew was okay and being looked after by someone he loved, it would have been very 'me' to embark on a spur-of-the-moment adventure after a few glasses of bubbles.

What I didn't know was that there was a reason why Tim had suddenly turned into the drink police. For months, he and Barry had been planning my *This Is Your Life* appearance, and it was going to be happening after the car show. Meanwhile, what Tim didn't know was that I wasn't feeling 100 per cent. It wasn't so bad that I needed to cancel – and I wouldn't have thought twice about cancelling an appearance at a car show if I'd been really ill – but I was feeling unwell enough to want a drink at Earl's Court, and not just in a social way.

Tim was very protective over me and made sure I didn't drink, which worked in my favour in one way, but not in another. Okay, I wouldn't be drunk for the show later, but neither could I calm my racing heart. By the time we got on the train back to Manchester, I was feeling poorly and anxious.

As we walked up the train corridor to our seats, I was surprised to see Barry and my other agent, Lindsay, coming towards us. 'What are you doing here?' I asked.

'We're going to see a play in Manchester,' they mumbled.

'That's nice,' I said dully.

My life was so ridiculous at the time that I had a double booking that day and had to then go – or so I thought – straight to open a garden centre in Bolton on the way home, and I didn't question that Tim was coming with me. 'Are you not going to redo your lipstick?' he asked me.

'Oh for goodness sake,' I snapped. 'Are you not bothered about me at all? I'm feeling terrible and I've got to go and open a garden centre!'

'Why not freshen up a bit?' he gently pressed.

I can't remember if I put some lipstick on. It's all a blur. Then the most nightmarish thing happened. The train drew in to Manchester, where a car would be picking us up and taking us to the garden centre in Bolton. As I got off the train, longing to be on my own, I saw a guy walking backwards in my direction holding a hand-held camera.

I was very famous at the time, so I assumed it was some punter making a sneaky video of me. 'Can you ask him not to do that?' I said to Tim.

A woman appeared and said, 'Denise Welch?'

'Yes,' I replied, caught by surprise.

She smiled. 'Your car is this way, round here.'

'Round where?' I thought.

Feeling like death, I followed her into an unknown (to me) corner of the station to find a massive great big stretch limousine waiting. As she opened the limo door, I said incredulously, 'A stretch limousine? To go to the Bolton Garden Centre?'

Everything seemed wrong; I didn't know what planet I was on. And things got a lot weirder when a grinning Michael Aspel jumped out of the limousine, holding the red book, and said the famous words, 'Denise Welch, this is your life!'

People I've spoken to who have done *This Is Your Life* say that this is a very surreal moment. Well, it was even more so for me, being in such a dark place to begin with. I had watched *This Is Your Life* as a child and always dreamt of being the subject of it, so it was sad that my dream came true when I was in that state. I felt awful. I did not know what was happening. And suddenly there was Michael Aspel in the back of a limousine.

Tim was also feeling the pressure, knowing how poorly I was. Fortunately, my acting skills kicked in automatically and I was able to show delighted surprise and all the rest of it, while silently trying to calculate how long it would be until the whole thing was over and I could go home to bed. Having done Tim's *This Is Your Life* the previous year, I knew that it would be hours and hours.

'I can't handle this, I can't handle this, I can't handle this,' I thought, my mind racing ahead. 'Who is going to be there? Who is not going to be there? I won't know half the people. How long will the night go on for?'

By the time I went into make-up at the studios I was almost monosyllabic, while trying to be somebody who was excited about what was happening. There was a big bunch of flowers waiting for me, but no wine in sight: Tim had obviously told the make-up people not to give me a drink, or maybe it was a general rule not to. After people like Oliver Reed had so disastrously taken advantage of hospitality before they went on programmes like Michael Aspel's chat show, *Aspel & Company*, the TV companies probably had a duty of care not to let you drink a lot.

I kept asking Ellie, the make-up artist, how much longer it would be until I went on set, all the while thinking: 'Oh my God, oh my God, oh my God.'

It was an ordeal having to sit in the chair and close my eyes to have my make-up applied. 'Get on with it. Get on with it. Get on with it,' I thought. I was jumping up every five minutes, saying, 'Sorry, I really need the toilet.'

In the toilets, I would stare at my reflection, thinking, 'I need a drink. I need a drink. I need a drink to take the pain away.'

When I eventually walked out in front of the studio audience and my completely ridiculous, surreal *This Is Your Life* experience began to unfold, all I could think was, 'I can't wait for this bit to be over and to go to the party, so that I can have a drink.'

And that's exactly what I did, so of course I felt terrible the next day.

It was such a shame, because it was an amazing thing to be on *This Is Your Life*, especially as I was the 1,000th person to appear. At least my acting got me through and nobody had any idea of what was happening to me internally. It was a huge thing to survive without having a complete breakdown. I was amazed I managed it. Afterwards, it felt as if I'd gone ten rounds with Mike Tyson (and, although I hadn't been able to knock him out, I had definitely won on points).

The postscript to this story is that a few days later I flew to Los Angeles to do a shoot for *HELLO!* magazine. So when my godfather, Ian La Frenais, came on as my final *This Is Your Life* guest – the all-important guest I hadn't seen for a long time, who they had flown all the way from Los Angeles for an emotional reunion – I whispered to him onstage, 'You know I'm coming out there in a couple of days, don't you?'

Magazines like *HELLO!* used to take people on really fabulous holidays to do photoshoots, and Tim and I, with Matthew, who was nine, went to Los Angeles for a fortnight and stayed at the Chateau Marmont. It was fantastic, especially as my 'From The Rovers to Rodeo Drive' shoot only took a couple of days and the rest of the time was ours.

Just recently, I happened to ask Ian La Frenais, 'When did you give up smoking?'

'You made me give up smoking,' he said.

'I did?'

'After *This Is Your Life*,' he said. 'I have never seen anybody smoke as much as you and Tim, and it made me give up.'

'I don't think I ever chain-smoked, though,' I said.

'Well, I remember you sitting at a Hollywood party I took you to, and you were drinking like a fish and lighting one cigarette after another,' he said.

I don't recall it, but I can believe it, because it was only a few days after *This Is Your Life* – and when I was in that surreal world of anxiety and depression, I did everything to excess.

III

When people ask me, 'Did you get ill after having Louis?', I want to say that I never stopped being ill after having Matthew. To this day, I still have depressive episodes, because that is my illness. At the same time, one of the reasons I hadn't got pregnant again in the years after Matthew was my fear of being as blackly, horribly ill with post-natal depression again. Another was that Tim didn't want another child, partly because of his age – he was coming up to fifty – and partly because of his understandable fear of losing his wife again, as he put it. Obviously we are delighted that we had Louis – of course we are – but that's why there was a twelve-year gap between my children.

I didn't make a conscious decision to get pregnant at forty-two; I didn't think there was any likelihood of it. Was I lax about precautions? Possibly, but although I think there was something in my body clock telling me that if I was going to do it, I had to do it now, I knew it was highly unlikely, bordering on the ridiculous, that doing it once in a month would result in the birth of a second child. And yet once did turn out to be enough – I got pregnant on a trip to Amsterdam with Tim. I was quietly excited when I found out, although worried about getting poorly. I had to have an amnio because I was an old mum, but everything was fine and I was really happy when I discovered I was having a boy at my 20-week scan.

I could trace my desire for a second child back seven years to the night my sister, Debbie, and I had drunk brandy together while we talked through Mum's initial decision to refuse a life-saving operation. My need for a sibling had been very strong during Mum's illness. It felt really important to have someone who understood exactly what I was going through, and vice versa, so I felt that it would be great for Matthew to have a brother.

I had a wonderful pregnancy with Louis – as I'd had with Matthew – and the reason for this was that my body was producing excessive oestrogen. Joy to the world, I don't remember once being depressed or anxious in the entire nine months of the pregnancy. I had an incredible gynaecologist in Gordon Faulkner, who was also one of my very close friends. Gordon suggested that I had an elective C-section, so that everything about the birth would be different to the first time. Nobody knew whether the original birth experience had any bearing on what had happened afterwards, but why not take the opportunity to do something different, since it was there? Gordon thought it would help to erase old scars if we made it a more pleasurable, controlled experience. It wasn't about being too posh to push; it was about taking control.

Gordon was more concerned about my mental health than anything else. 'Don't you worry if you have a couple of glasses of wine,' he said. 'You've got no idea of the Vinegar Veras that I treat. Some of them are at the vodka from morning to night!'

He was clearly making up these other boozy patients to make me laugh, while at the same time saying, 'It is much better that you don't get anxious, and that you stay well. Don't worry about having the odd glass of wine. You'll be fine.'

I did drink a little bit when I was pregnant, but only like other people drink when they're pregnant: a glass of wine, here and there. I never got drunk and had no need to self-medicate my depression, because I felt fantastic, mentally and physically.

Tim and I were a bit worried when it came to telling Matthew about the baby. Matthew had been a very happy only child for twelve years; he was never a kid who desperately wanted a sibling, because we always made sure that he had a pal with him when we went away on holiday or went out as a family. This was wonderful in a way, because it meant that he had someone to play with, but didn't fight with! He was very close to his cousins too, so he was always 'only, not lonely' as a child. Thankfully, he wasn't upset when we said we were having a baby. He asked if he could have an orangutan instead, but then accepted that a baby was the only option on the table, apart from a scooter.

At the scans, everything had shown as normal, so I knew I was giving birth to a healthy child. Yet the night before my C-section, I couldn't stop my mind swirling with worry. Would I be ill afterwards? Would the baby be okay? Would I be able to love him as much as I loved Matthew? I couldn't imagine loving anyone as much as I loved Matthew.

The C-section at Hope Hospital wasn't a walk in the park, but it was a lot better than forty-two hours of labour without painkillers.

'Bloomin' 'eck, it's like a shopping bag!' Tim said, referring to the foetal sac, as he watched Gordon in action behind the surgeon's screen. It was now traditional for him to say something intensely annoying at the very moment I was giving birth.

And suddenly, there was sweet little Louis, my gorgeous baby, weighing in at a healthy 7lb 3oz! Tim and I were over the moon. Before long, Mum and Dad and Matthew came in to see us, followed by my friend Rose, who was pregnant and soon to have Harrison, who would become Louis's lifelong friend.

Everything was blissful, with one exception. I desperately wanted to breastfeed Louis, but every time I tried, he wasn't latching on for long enough to get any milk. His blood sugars were fine – the nurses weren't concerned – but I was upset and couldn't help worrying that he wasn't getting the nutrients he needed.

Meanwhile, Tim was thrilled to have Louis and delighted that I hadn't plunged into depression.

I was quietly hopeful that I would be okay, but: 'It's early days yet,' I cautioned.

On our third day in hospital, I was on my own in my room with a midwife, trying out another feeding position with Louis, when he suddenly vomited up a jet of liquid the colour of the greenest bile. It was like a scene out of *Alien*, or *The Exorcist*.

'Okay, I think we'll just pop him down to special care,' the midwife said calmly.

My stomach turned over. 'What's the matter with him?' I asked.

'Oh, it could be a variety of things, but don't you worry,' she said breezily. 'They'll sort him out in special care.'

Despite her calm manner, I couldn't help panicking. As they were getting Louis ready to be taken down, I went into the toilet and started breathing deeply to stem my anxiety. Through the open door, I could see Eamonn Holmes's face on the television. 'Please don't come!' I told the unwelcome visitor. 'If there is any time in my life you cannot come, it's to this hospital now, because my baby needs me. I might lose my child! You cannot come to this ward.'

Three days earlier, I'd thought I'd had a healthy baby. Now I had a very sick baby and nobody knew what was the matter with him. If my depression were to come on for psychological reasons, this would be a prime moment for it. I was worried out of my wits about Louis and terrified that I would get ill too.

Louis was in the special care unit for two weeks, encased in an incubator, with wires and tubes coming out of him. He couldn't keep anything down, so he was being fed through a tube in his tummy. Meanwhile the nurses kept trying to give him tiny amounts of milk using syringes. I was allowed to take him out of his incubator, all wired up, and sit with him on my knee. My heart used to race as I held him. 'Don't let this become anxiety!' I'd tell myself.

'This is just normal stress and worry,' I kept repeating silently. 'It's normal anxiety.'

I spent a lot of that time warding off the unwelcome visitor. It took up a huge reserve of energy. I was sleeping very sparsely, never for more than two hours at a stretch, and every time I woke up, I'd panic, thinking, 'Is he here? Is he here? Is he here? Am I all right? Am I all right? Am I all right? Okay, okay, okay. I'm all right. I'm all right. I'm all right. I'm dealing with this like a normal person, like a proper mum.'

The special care unit was downstairs from the maternity ward, at the end of a very long corridor that I called the 'green mile' because it seemed to get longer and longer as I walked it, dreading the thought of being given bad news when I reached the end.

I would buzz on the door and say, 'Hello, it's Denise, Louis's mum,' or 'It's Mrs Healy,' and wait in trepidation for their response. I could tell by the tone of their voice if it was good or bad.

'Come in, Denise!' I'd hear.

I'd go in and they'd say, 'He's taken a tiny syringe of milk!' and we would be celebrating.

Or they'd say, 'We've taken him for a lumbar puncture. It's not meningitis.'

There were days when I'd buzz and say, 'Hello, it's Denise,' and they'd respond flatly: 'Come in, Mrs Healy.'

My heart would be racing. 'Why is the voice like that?' I'd think.

When I got in, I'd be told, 'He threw the milk up again.'

They seemed to be getting no nearer to finding out what was wrong with Louis. Whatever it was, it was very serious. Every day, it was, 'Well, it's not meningitis, it's not Crohn's disease and it's not . . .'

After two weeks, I was at my wits' end. 'Please, please, please, tell me what it is, not what it isn't,' I begged.

They decided to send Louis to Alder Hey Hospital, a surgical hospital, where the doctors did another round of tests and biopsies. After ruling out a twisted bowel, they began to suspect that Louis might have something called Hirschsprung's disease, which occurs in one in five thousand babies; it's when the nerve endings in the bowel haven't formed normally during the first trimester of pregnancy. I got the sense that if it wasn't Hirschsprung's, the doctors were stumped as to other possibilities, so I started hoping it was, even though it would mean surgery for little Louis.

Although we lived only about an hour by car from Alder Hey, I felt a strong need to be near Louis night and day; I couldn't bear the idea of leaving the hospital to go home. If they had let me, I would have slept in a chair by his cot. Instead, I was lucky enough to stay in the Ronald McDonald Children's Charities house, which provides people with a place to stay when their children are being treated at the hospital. It was a lifesaver for me: it meant I could see Louis as soon as he woke up in the morning and put him to bed at night.

I felt guilty about being away from Matthew, because I had originally told him that I'd go into hospital, have the baby and come back a few days later. Of course things hadn't worked out that way and he was coming in to see me and Louis in the hospital with Tim almost every day. Although I made sure to cuddle Matthew, love him and reassure him, he would snuggle into the bed with me while I was holding Louis and try to get in between us. 'Matthew, watch the baby! Matthew, don't!' I'd chide.

After the nurses taught Tim and me how to feed Louis and give him enemas, we were allowed to take him home while we waited for the results of all his biopsies. Bless him, we had to feed him and then pull a little poo out of his bottom using a tube, so it was a very odd time. Yet I didn't get an episode of depression, even though you can't be more anxious than when you're faced with the possibility of losing your child.

Two weeks later, the hospital rang and confirmed that Louis had Hirschsprung's disease. I was relieved, because at last they had found out what was wrong with him, and it was treatable, even though it meant that at just six weeks old he would have to be operated on. Later I found out that the first successful Hirschsprung's operation was done in 1948, just ten years before I was born. Prior to then, Louis would have been 'a child who didn't thrive', as my granny would have put it, a thought that makes me shudder to this day. We were incredibly lucky that there were three research projects on Hirschsprung's being conducted at Alder Hey, and that one of the world's top Hirschsprung's surgeons, Graham Lamont, was based there.

A couple of days before Louis's operation, he went back into hospital for pre-surgery preparation. I found it difficult to leave Matthew again, knowing that he desperately wanted me to be at home. I must have mentioned it to the doctors at Alder Hey because after a few hours at the hospital, they said, 'Why don't you go home, spend the evening with Matthew, get a good night's sleep and come back tomorrow? There's nothing spoiling here. We'll call you if there's a problem.'

I took their advice and when I got home, I sat with Tim and Matthew, watching TV. But however hard I tried, I couldn't be present in the room. It was as if I was attached by an umbilical cord to Louis, and it was pulling me to him. It was the weirdest feeling, an impulse I couldn't stop. Even though I knew my eldest son wanted me to stay home, I had to go back to the hospital.

'Darling,' I said to Matthew, 'I am so sorry. Your brother will be home soon, but I have to go to him and be with him while he's in hospital. You will have me back, but right now, he needs me more than you do.'

'It's all right, Mum,' Matthew said.

I drove back to the hospital in floods of tears and didn't leave again until Louis had had the operation and we finally got him home. It was a tough time and I had a lot of guilt about Matthew, so I was very coiled and wound, but only in the same way that any mother would have been.

I was grateful to the unwelcome visitor for not coming. I didn't thank him, because I hate the unwelcome visitor – he's blighted my life and he's blighted the lives of those who love me – but I was grateful that he'd stayed away when my child needed me.

The next time I had an episode, it came as randomly as ever and wasn't related to any event or circumstance. That's why it didn't make sense to me when psychologists talked about the psychological aspects of post-natal depression and dismissed my belief that it was hormonal. You know your own body – and if there was any time and place that depression was going to come through the door, it was through the door of that hospital.

It's a strange irony that when Matthew was born, he was a healthy, bouncing baby of 8lbs and I was plunged into a deep, dark depression, whereas when Louis was born, he was a terribly, terribly sick baby and yet I wasn't plunged into that same blackness. I was emotionally traumatised by what was happening to my son, but I didn't get clinical depression while he was in the hospital or in special care.

Considering everything that went on in those first few weeks of Louis's life, I can't believe how calm I was throughout it all. Something kicked in – a coping mechanism – and it kicked in again when Louis was twenty months old and we came within an hour of losing him due to adhesions caused by the operation he'd had at six weeks.

I had brought on my illness many times by thinking, 'Wouldn't it be awful if I got ill?' but neither time Louis was ill did it come. Yes, I continued to have episodes of depression, but only in the same way as I had for the previous twelve years.

IV

My aunties and their friends in Whitley Bay thought there was no role greater than being the landlady of the Rovers Return. No matter whether you went on to do seventeen films with Al Pacino, leaving that role voluntarily could only mean one thing – you had completely lost your marbles. Which of course I had!

When I left *Coronation Street* in 2000, I was pregnant with Louis and couldn't have been happier. Even though people said I was crazy, I was sure I wanted to leave. Nevertheless, you do worry when you voluntarily leave a soap whether you'll ever work again, so it was encouraging to get a job soon afterwards, in a series starring James Bolam, Michael French and Jenna Russell.

Set in the 1950s and filmed in the village of Downham in Lancashire, *Born and Bred* was a light-hearted comedy drama. The producer, Phil Collinson, cast me as Edie, a recurring character, because he wanted to see me do something outside of being the buxom blonde (although I wasn't so buxom at the time, because I was so thin). Edie had six children and I played her wearing no make-up, with hair scraped back and dowdy 1950s clothes. It was a fantastic role for me to have after *Coronation Street* because it was so different.

Very often, my memories of life are tainted by recalling the moments I got ill, but *Born and Bred* shines in my memory and I don't remember ever being ill while I was doing it. I loved it and it's a joy to look back on. Every day of filming is a sunny day in my memory, perhaps because it was such a pleasurable time.

Soon afterwards, when Louis was six months old, I appeared in an episode of *The Vice*, a drama series about the Metropol-itan Police vice unit starring Ken Stott. In this episode, I was a guest lead with Peter Firth; Peter's character was running a high-class prostitute ring and I was his long-suffering wife. It was a great role and we had a lovely director in Tim Leandro. When the episode aired, a couple of my friends said they were moved to tears by a scene that focused on my facial expression as I was taking my make-up off at the end of an evening, while my husband was very audibly having sex with someone else in the next room.

Peter and I were meant to be the owners of a mansion in Hertfordshire worth £20 million, where we filmed many of our scenes. One day, while we were between shots, Peter and some of the other guys were watching TV in the conservatory. I was in the front room talking to the director when we heard one of the guys say, 'What the . . . ?'

'What is it?' we asked, making our way over.

The guys in the conservatory all had a look on their faces like I'd never seen before. I glanced over at the television and saw the second plane hit the World Trade Center. It was 11 September 2001 and New York was under attack.

Like everybody else watching, as soon as that plane went into that building, I knew the world had changed. Everything in the atmosphere was different from that moment on. Nobody could believe what was happening. The screen was filled with images of people running through the streets of New York, screaming.

We didn't know what to do. We stood around in a state of shock until Tim Leandro said, 'We're going to have to carry on, guys.'

'What is happening? Surely we're not going to go on filming?' I thought, in a panic.

It was the same weird feeling I had the day Princess Diana died and we did the scene in 'Firman's Freezers'. I looked around the room to check that everyone was dealing with it in the same way I was.

'But we don't know what is happening!' someone said.

'No, we don't know what is happening, but we are going to have to continue,' Tim said, more firmly.

We went back to work. Every time Tim said, 'Cut!' we ran to the television to see the latest developments – and things were getting worse and worse.

Later, we had to do an exterior shot outside Ken Stott's character's flat in east London. Everything felt surreal. One of the cameramen kept saying, 'There's going to be a war.'

I could feel my heart racing. 'Don't say that!' I pleaded.

'If it's a terror attack, there will be a war,' he said.

While Ken Stott and I were outside the flat having a fag break, we looked through the glass frontage of a wine bar and saw people drinking and having what looked like a normal night, seemingly oblivious to the live coverage from New York on the television in the corner. 'Why are they just laughing with their friends?' I thought. 'Don't they feel the way I do about what has happened?'

I was incredulous that normal life was going on while the world was changing. I could feel my illness coming on and by the time we wrapped, I was in a complete state. It was another example of how being gripped by fear and panic could set off a chemical reaction in my body and bring on my illness, but this time, unusually, it was caused by world events.

'Are you all right?' Tim asked, as we were leaving.

'No,' I said.

'Would you like to come home and stay with me and my wife tonight?'

'No,' I thought. 'I need to have a drink.' Out loud, I lied: 'That's really kind of you, thank you, but I've got a friend coming round to my hotel. Honestly, I'll be fine.'

I went back to my hotel and had a couple of drinks before falling exhausted into bed. It upset me to see the next morning that one of the red-top papers had changed its banner to black. 'THE DAY THE WORLD CHANGED', ran the headline. I sat in bed, feeling anxious and jittery.

That evening, my friend Lester tried to persuade me to meet him at a wine bar in Knightsbridge. 'I don't want to. I can't. I've got my thing,' I told him.

'But you need to be with people at a time like this,' he said. 'We all do.'

He was right, but the only way to be around people was to try to numb my illness with alcohol, and once I was at the wine bar with Lester and the others, I decided to get hammered. I had been living a very moderate life since Louis had been born, but 9/11 had really knocked me and I wanted to self-medicate how I was feeling.

While I was in the ladies, a beautiful young woman came up to me and said, 'Oh my God, you're my favourite actress! You're amazing! I love you!'

'Thank you,' I said, flattered. 'Isn't this awful, what's happened in New York? I don't even know why I'm here. I just feel I need to be with people.'

'Are you tying one on tonight?' she asked.

'Well, I'm filming tomorrow, but I've only got one tiny driving scene with no dialogue, so I don't care if I get drunk,' I said.

'Can I come and join you? I'm on my own,' she said.

This surprised me. 'You're on your own?'

'Yes, my friends have left.'

'Absolutely! Come over and meet my friends!' I offered, taking her arm.

That's how we bonded. Later, she opened up about her life: her name was Myra; she came from a wealthy but complicated family; she had an apartment in a smart area of London and a boat on the Thames. I don't know now how much of this was true, but at the time I had no reason to disbelieve her. It didn't occur to me that she might be a journalist.

During the four weeks that Myra was trying to catch me out and get a story on me, she probably rang me about twenty times. She was always asking me to meet her at a bar, or go with her to this party or that nightclub event. I didn't accept any of her invitations because, as she must have been very aware, I was too busy living my normal, respectable, working-mum's life in the north, with my baby and twelve-year-old son.

Now, Myra could talk, and I was sympathetic when she told me about the problems she was having with her family. I tried to make room for her, even though I was busy and didn't really know her, because I felt sorry for her and she seemed to have very few friends or people she could confide in. However, being a working mum meant that I often didn't have a minute to spare, so I was always saying, 'I'm going to have to cut you off there because I've got to go and get Matthew from school,' or 'Hi Myra, I'm just going to bath Louis; can I ring you back another time?' or 'I'm just going on set for *Soap Fever*, Myra; I can't talk now.'

This was how it was for all but one of the calls I had from Myra. The last time, I was in Spain doing a photoshoot and was alone in the apartment we had there, when the call came through. 'I'm having a party next week. Would you like to come?' Myra said.

I happened to be free on the day and said I would try to make it. A few minutes after I'd put the phone down, she called again, asking if it would bother me if people were taking cocaine at the party. 'No,' I said, laughing. 'I wouldn't be shocked or offended, don't worry.'

'Do you take it?' she asked.

'I used to,' I said. 'Now it's only on high days and holidays.'

'You don't know anyone who could get me some, do you?'

'No, I don't,' I said, racking my brains. 'But I could maybe make a couple of calls and see if I can get you a number.'

'Great,' she said.

The following weekend, the *Sunday Mirror* ran a front-page story about my 'cocaine use'. It turned out that Myra was the cousin of Mazher Mahmood, the undercover reporter known as 'the fake sheikh', and she had been taping our conversations for a month, because it took her that long to get anything remotely incriminating out of me.

For years afterwards, I assumed that Myra had simply been an opportunist; that it was my bad luck that a journalist happened to be in the toilets that night, and that she had grabbed the chance to hang around, befriend me and stitch me up. It wasn't until years later, when I was sorting out my hacking case against the *Mirror*, that I discovered that Myra had been sent to the bar to meet me. She knew I was going to be there because my phone had been hacked by the *Mirror*, as it continued to be hacked for years to come, sowing seeds of paranoia and distrust in my life that led me and my visitor down a very dark path.

V

Mostly my depression is exactly that – depression. But when I started working on my next TV series, *Down To Earth*, in 2004, I experienced a long period of pure anxiety. For a whole year, I woke up in the mornings to a pounding heart and a feeling of such gasping panic that I couldn't swallow properly. Every morning felt like the night of my first panic attack after I had Matthew. The strange thing was that I wasn't anxious about anything specific. There was nothing I could relate it to. It felt very physical, as if something was going on in my system that I had no control over.

Down To Earth was a comedy drama set in a Devon village. Ricky Tomlinson and I were co-leads and our characters owned the village pub. I was thrilled to get the job and didn't let on to anyone that I was in an almost perpetual state of anxiety. It was very tough going at times. I was having an especially bad day when I went down to London for the first cast read-through. Sitting at the long table, looking around at a room full of actors that included Ricky and Bernard Cribbins, I felt like a swan on the water, with its legs going manically underneath. Yet I had no reason to feel anxious, because I could still do the read-through standing on my head. My body was out of control in a way that didn't relate to anything that was going on in my mind.

I remember being introduced to Bernard Cribbins, who was going to play my dad. We used to call Bernard and Ricky the 'Chuckle Brothers' because they never stopped with their jokes, and that day I had my first taste of Bernard's high-spirited personality. I tried to laugh along, but actually my heart was racing, and I wanted to scream: 'You've got no idea what I'm going through!'

One of Tim's cousins was getting married around this time. Matthew was going to be an usher and Louis a little flower boy. It shows how mentally ill I was that I was unable to go. My anxiety was so great that I couldn't get out of bed without being sick – and nobody wants a shaking, sweating, vomiting relative at their wedding, no matter what they say about it not being the same without you.

I was very grateful that Tim and the boys understood that I was ill and couldn't come, but when I look at the photos of that day now, it still upsets me that I missed seeing my children take part in such a special family occasion. You can't get those moments back. Eventually, I had to take very strong beta blockers to keep my anxiety at bay.

When my depression came on during *Down To Earth*, it was mostly grey depression, which meant I could go through the motions and still pull out a good performance. But there was one day when it came on so black and thick that my mouth started to twist and I found it hard to enunciate my words.

We were filming an interior scene at the pub Ricky and I owned. 'Are you all right, Den?' asked Zara Dawson, who was playing my daughter.

'No,' I said.

Zara reached over and gripped my hand. I've never forgotten it. She was only twenty-one but she possessed empathy beyond her years.

There was a car parked outside the pub that belonged to Jackie, my character. 'Have you got the keys for the car?' I asked the props guy.

'Yes,' he said.

'Can I have them?'

'Why?'

'Can I just hold them?' I said.

He looked at me as if I was crazy, which I guess I was. I didn't explain that I needed to know I had an escape route, in the same way I needed to know how to flee the theatre when I was onstage. I needed the car keys in my pocket to reassure me, because I felt so bad that I kept thinking, 'I can't do this! I'm going to run out of here, get in the car, drive off and nobody will be able to find me.'

After I'd got through the scene, my depression started to lift, thankfully. Every time the visitor leaves, it gives me strength for the next time. 'He's gone, I've won!' I think jubilantly. 'See? If I can get through that with you there, I can get through anything,' I tell him.

This has become one of my mantras. Later, when I watched the episode and that scene, I could see the depression in my eyes, but nobody else would have been able to tell.

I hated letting anyone down, illness or not, especially the people I loved. At least my nearest and dearest understood my depression, but I was aware that audiences and critics might not, and I was always very fearful of going onstage when the unwelcome visitor was at my door. If he was wearing his grey cloak, I could just about work through it, but when he arrived wearing his black cloak, it was nigh on impossible to do anything – although occasionally, I had to bite the bullet and carry on regardless.

In late 2004, I signed up to do a pantomime in Stockport. It had been a busy year, which had begun with my return to the theatre after seven years away. In January, I'd played the character of Mari Hoff, Little Voice's boozy, brassy mum, in *The Rise and Fall of Little Voice* at one of my favourite theatres, the Manchester Royal Exchange. The play had been a sell-out, the reviews were amazing and I received two awards for my performance.

After that, I'd gone off to Devon to film *Down To Earth*, where I had a much-publicised affair with the set carpenter, who sold a story to the papers after it ended. This prompted Tim and me to re-evaluate our marriage, which wasn't great by this point. Over the years, there had been infidelities on both sides of the marriage. We spent a lot of time apart working and when we were at home we compounded our problems with our drinking. I now realise that we were self-medicating our marriage, although neither of us realised it, maybe because we were also enabling each other to drink. And I'm not sure if we really thought we had a choice about splitting up, because our lives were so entwined and enmeshed. We were bringing up our sons together, we loved each other's families, had masses of shared friends and a public profile as a couple. We decided to stay together.

I took the job in Stockport because the theatre was on my doorstep and I wanted to stay close to home and family after the emotional turbulence of recent times. I didn't really want to do a pantomime, but they pay very well. Still, I never seem to have much luck with them.

My very first experience of doing a pantomime was *Jack and the Beanstalk* in Bury St Edmunds in 1986, when I got the flu, fainted while I was halfway up the beanstalk and ended up in hospital with pleurisy!

Years later, after my depression had come on, I was doing *Jack and the Beanstalk* again, this time at the Newcastle Theatre Royal. It was a big pantomime with a lot of money invested in it. In the main, at the time, I was okay. My sister and her family were now living at the Hemmel and I was staying with them, travelling back to Stocksfield every night after the show.

One night, I was onstage, just about to go into a speech about a perm. Now, a poem, in Geordie, is pronounced 'a perm', and my line was, 'I went in the hairdresser's and said,

"Can I have a perm?" And she said, "Aye, Mary had a little lamb . . ."'

Seconds before I was to say these words, I got my whoosh. I managed to say, 'I went in the hairdresser's and said, "Can I have a perm?" . . .' and then everything went black.

The next thing I knew, the curtain was coming down and I was on the floor with a crowd around me. It was the most horrible feeling. 'Do you think you can go back on?' people were asking.

'I can't remember anything,' I said groggily.

Someone got me a glass of water and people rubbed my shoulders and forehead to calm me down. 'Okay, I can go back on now,' I said.

Fogwell Flax, the comedian, who was also in the show, said, 'It's all right, I know your lines. I'll get you through it.'

The curtain went back up and the audience applauded. Suddenly I was in this parallel universe, onstage with words coming out of my mouth, silently panicking about running off. By the time the show ended, I was shaking and crying.

So, pantomimes weren't my favourite thing to do, and now I was playing the Wicked Queen in a production of *Snow White* at the Plaza Theatre in Stockport. We only had a week's rehearsal, which is a ridiculously short time to stage a full-scale show, but not uncommon in the pantomime world. Cutting things even finer, on the fourth day of rehearsals they were allowing me to have the afternoon off to go to the *Manchester Evening News* Theatre Awards, where I had been nominated for Best Actress.

I was fine and dandy that day, not in a million years thinking I'd win, and off I went to Manchester. When I arrived, I was surprised to see Mum and Dad, as I had no idea that they were going to be there. Needless to say, because they were there, I won the Best Actress award. For me, it was like winning an Olivier. I'd won *TV Quick* awards, and I'd been up for

'Sexiest Soap Female' and all these different things over the years, but this felt like a grown-up award. I'm not dismissing the other awards, which were hugely flattering, but to win a theatre award for a performance with the Royal Exchange Theatre Company was really massive for me.

The award was presented to me by Brian Conley. I had heard that Brian had given up drinking and asked how it was going. Brian was on top form and happy to tell me how brilliant he felt, but did I listen? No: after the awards I went with Tim to the after-party in Manchester and had too much to drink, fully aware that I only had another four days of rehearsals to go before we opened with *Snow White*.

In the morning, I woke up feeling really, really anxious. I felt furious with myself that I had potentially helped bring anxiety on by drinking. As I was driving back to work, I got it into my mind that the rest of the cast would know that I had won a Best Actress award, and the audiences would also know. What, then, if I couldn't pull off my performance as the Wicked Queen?

I imagined everyone thinking, 'How did she win that "Best Actress" award, because she's *terrible* in this pantomime!'

By the time I got to work I was having a huge panic attack, convinced that my bleak vision would come true. The previous day, I'd been absolutely fine. Now I'd ruined everything, just as I was about to open in the show, by drinking too much and inducing anxiety that was fast turning into depression.

The first night of *Snow White* was horrendous. My visitor arrived, wearing a black cloak, and was beside me during my first speech, which was a long monologue. Gripped by depression, I dried halfway through and had to walk off and look to the stage manager for my lines. It makes me feel ill now when I think of it. Back then, the Plaza Theatre was a really depressing place with an old organ that rose out of the floor. Every song that was played on that organ sounded like the theme tune of a horror film, which just made things worse.

Backstage, I tried to appear okay, because we had lots of little kids in the show and the last thing I wanted was for them to worry about how their leading lady was. Normally in a panto, I would spend time with the cast and throw a party for 'the babes', as they're known, but now I was coming offstage and going straight to my dressing room. The only person I confided in was Davinia, who dressed me and helped me through several lavish costume changes. I shall always be grateful to Davinia for her understanding and support.

When you start doing a show, you often play little japes onstage to make each other corpse, especially in pantomimes. In this production, Snow White had a basket, and the rest of the cast were putting rude things in it to surprise her. I laughed along with the joke, and wished I felt well enough to join in. The 'normal me' would have got something rude from Ann Summers and popped it in the basket when she wasn't looking, but getting to the shops was out of the question, just then – it was enough of a struggle to get dressed in the morning.

When I have a really serious depression and the visitor is in a black cloak, rather than a grey cloak, I can't eat anything. This is why, when I was first poorly after Matthew, I lost two stone in three weeks. Now, I wasn't eating again. Mum and Dad were staying with us and Mum tried to make me sip meal replacement drinks, but even those were difficult to swallow.

'But you've got to eat something,' people kept saying.

I tried. I would go to Greggs and buy something naughty but delicious that I really loved, like a steak slice, or a cheese pasty. Then I'd sit in my dressing room and try to eat it without retching. But it didn't matter how tasty it was, it was like putting sandpaper in my mouth. I started to avoid food altogether, telling my family that I was eating at the theatre, and Davinia that I had eaten before I'd come in.

The days went on, just getting through it, every day frozen before I went onstage, thinking that I couldn't remember the lines because I'd dried the first time. Every night, I drove back through the darkness and tried not to have a drink when I got home. Each morning, as I was driving back to the theatre for the matinee, I thought about crashing the car so that I wouldn't have to go on. I didn't want to have a fatal crash, or even to injure myself, particularly – I just wanted to be taken to hospital so that I didn't have to do the show. Then everyone would feel sorry for me because I'd been in a car crash, and would understand why I'd had to pull out of the rest of the run.

Years later, I understood what Will Young had been going through when he dropped out of BBC TV's *Strictly Come Dancing* and said he had considered breaking his own leg so that he could get out of it for physical reasons, because he didn't want to say what he was going through mentally. I genuinely thought about crashing the car every day I was in *Snow White*. When the road was clear and I knew I wouldn't put anybody else in harm's way, I'd think, 'If I just turned the wheel now . . .'

Something held me back, though.

As I drove home from the theatre on Christmas Eve, I tried to think positively. 'When I wake up tomorrow, it will have gone,' I told myself.

When I walked into the house, my sister was crying. Tim said, 'Come here, flower,' and gave me a cuddle. It turned out that Sadie, our beloved boxer dog, had choked on a stick and died. It was such a fluke accident that my brain couldn't take it in.

Christmas was horrendous. All my family came down and we went out to a pub. Feeling weird, I went through the motions, but couldn't feel a thing.

My lovely friend Lisa, who was Louis's nanny at the time, popped in with her mum and dad. 'You look really thin. You're not well, are you?' she said to me, looking concerned.

'No, I'm all right. I'm fine. I'm fine. I'm fine,' I said.

When I went back to work on Boxing Day, I was at the theatre when the news broke that there had been an earthquake and tsunami in the Indian Ocean, and that hundreds of thousands of people had died as a result. I was panicked and appalled when I heard the stories of horror, drowning and death. They plunged me into a state of paranoia and I started to think that everybody I knew was going to die.

Something had happened in the universe: Sadie was the start of it; the tsunami was next. Now everybody was going to die: my family, my children, everybody.

I went on to do the first half of the show. Back in the dressing room for my first costume change, I collapsed. All I remember is reaching out for Davinia as I fell, clutching onto the sink, and then nothing. I passed out.

'That's it! You need to go home. You can't go on again,' Davinia said when I came to.

I went back on. I had to. I remember sitting on my Wicked Queen's throne onstage, looking out at the audience and not quite knowing where I was. When I came off at the interval, Tim was in my dressing room. 'Davinia called and told me what happened,' he said. 'You're coming home with me.'

'I can't!' I protested. 'Please, let me go on.'

He shook his head. 'I'm taking you home.'

'Please, let me go on. We've got no understudy. I can't let them down.'

'No,' he said, helping me get undressed and into my clothes. 'She won't be coming back,' he told the stage manager.

Back at home, I lay in bed, tortured by guilt. How would the show continue? There was no Wicked Queen.

I didn't go back. Nobody died. It was a real lesson for me, because they got an actress in to read the Wicked Queen onstage for two days, by which time another actress had learned the part and the show went on.

Yet I was so poorly that I couldn't stop fretting about it. 'Please ring them up and find out if they all hate me!' I begged Tim.

He rang them. 'What did they say?' I asked him anxiously. 'Are they supportive? Are they sympathetic? Are they angry?'

The company were very nice about it, and the national papers were kind when they picked the story up a few days later. Not so the local Stockport newspaper, however, which reported that I had let down thousands of fans in the north-west by pulling out of a pantomime midway through, citing "nervous exhaustion", with those horrible inverted commas implying that I was making up an illness, or it was psycho-somatic, or the result of excess alcohol.

I winced as I read on that the actress playing Snow White had "saved the day" because, despite having a sprained wrist and wearing a pot plaster, she went on, ignoring the pain in her arm, and delivered a first-class performance to thousands of cheery children.

'Oh my God,' I thought as I read it, and the hurt has stayed with me ever since.

Of all the things that have been written about me, that piece in the Stockport paper has upset me the most. I've often quoted it when I've given mental health talks, because it high-lights how ignorant people can be. If the writer had only known what I would have given to continue in the show! I would have gone onstage even if I'd had a pot plaster covering my feet to my head, with only my eyes showing. Yet I was so, so poorly that I simply couldn't carry on. I hadn't eaten for three weeks. I had black, thick depression onstage. I barely knew who I was, let alone what I was saying.

The barbed comments in that article were heartbreaking for me. They really affected me badly and slowed down my recovery, because I was racked with worry about what people were thinking about me.

Our tribe, those with this illness, live with the mentality that the really brave people are the ones who carry on despite debilitating physical conditions. They are – my God, of course they are – but so are we.

I began to wonder why I went on drinking. It was a vicious circle. I was drinking to stop the depression, which was causing the depression. I'd wake up feeling poorly and hungover and spend my days wanting to have a drink again, to try to feel better.

Mum had given up drinking by then. She didn't like me drinking the way I did, but whenever she tried to talk to me about it, I'd say, 'I'm fine, don't worry about me! You'd drink too if you had my illness.'

I didn't only drink to feel better – I drank socially, too. But I couldn't drink like other people. Alcoholics can't, because there is no off-button. Things got progressively worse and I started to have blackouts. There were whole evenings when I could only remember my first couple of drinks – then, nothing. I had no recollection of where I'd been or what I'd done afterwards; I didn't even have flashbacks. I had to rely on people to tell me what had happened.

When my family tried to tackle me about it, I'd say the sort of things that I've subsequently in sobriety heard other people say to their loved ones to excuse their drinking.

'For God's sake, I'm working hard to keep this family together! Stop having a go at me! I need to let my hair down. You're all buzz-kills.'

Tim and I and the boys used to go on holiday to Turkey with a boozy bunch of pals we'd met through Matthew's school. Sometimes Mum and Dad came along as well, which was fantastic, as they got on with everybody and we loved having them. It was also quite useful, because if we went out in the evenings Mum was happy to stay at home in the villa and look after Louis, who was still quite little. The upside of this, for the alcoholic in me, was that I could tie one on if I wanted to, without having to worry. The downside of it was that I was already having a bad time with my depression, and drinking made it worse. It had taken a long time to recover from my breakdown during the Stockport pantomime and my periods of wellness were getting shorter.

In early 2005, about halfway through one of these holidays in Turkey, I went out with the crowd one evening. After dinner, I took Louis back to Mum. 'Go and enjoy yourself, but don't drink too much!' Mum called after me, as I left.

'I won't!' I yelled back.

I don't remember anything else about the evening. I woke up the next day with no recollection of it at all. Instead of memories of fun and laughter, I had a horrible hangover and depression. And, as usual, I hated myself for it. Hangovers make you anxious anyway and I had an added sense of self-loathing.

'Why can't I just go out and be a normal person and have a normal drink and then come home to bed?' I asked myself.

I got up and went into the lounge. Everything seemed strange; nothing seemed right and I had a strong desire to run away and never come back. But you can't escape your own head. It was very frightening.

Mum was out by the pool with Louis. I went to join them and immediately started crying because I felt so low. Within minutes my depression became so thick and black that I started to have a massive panic attack. 'I've got to go home!' I gasped, shaking and crying. 'I've got to stop drinking, I'm *going* to stop drinking, I've got to stop this.'

'Do whatever you need to do, pet,' Mum said, giving me a hug. 'I'll look after Louis. You go and sort yourself out.'

Tim said he would come home with me. I was grateful, but it also made me feel guilty that I was ruining everybody's holiday, even though everybody was telling me that I wasn't and they just wanted me to get well.

I don't remember the practicalities of what happened, but obviously Tim must have got me on a flight. When I got home, I phoned Kevin Kennedy, who played Curly Watts in *Coronation Street*. Kevin and I had struggled together with our alcohol dependency during our *Coronation Street* years.

Funnily enough, one of the things I remember about my terrible fortieth birthday party – the one when I was really depressed – is Clare Kennedy, Kevin's wife, bursting into tears and saying, 'I tried, Denise! I tried to come for you, but I've got to go now. In fact, Al-Anon has told me that I've got to leave Kevin altogether to show how serious his sobriety has to be.'

Al-Anon is a branch of Alcoholics Anonymous (AA) and offers a network of support groups throughout the world for people who need help coping with a problem drinker in their lives, or who have been affected by someone else's alcoholism. Going to Al-Anon taught Clare not to make idle threats. She had told Kevin she would leave the party if he was going to drink, and she did. Subsequently, she realised that she herself had alcohol problems and they've both just celebrated twenty years of being sober.

Now I had convinced myself that if I gave up drinking I would get well. I was desperate to not get ill again. Kevin came and got me and took me to my first AA meeting, in Cheshire, where I admitted for the first time that I had a drink problem. 'This is it, now. I'm going to be sober and well,' I thought, naively.

You are generally advised not to share your story at your first time at AA. It's better to listen and see how it works before you do. But I wanted to share my story, even though I could see Kevin looking over at me as if to say, 'No, don't do it.' It makes me cringe and go red, thinking about it now.

I was fascinated by the set-up of AA, because I'd never been before. Here were these strangers, all with something in common, telling their stories. One particular guy very confidently got up and described his descent into alcoholism. He told us how he had been the owner of an off-licence, but drank his own profits away; people would come in to buy a bottle of wine and find him slumped behind the till.

It was a rollercoaster of a story with upsetting parts and funny parts and, by the time he'd finished, I thought, 'Good for him!'

However, each time I went to the meeting, he told the same story again, which eventually made me want to reach for the vodka. I went half a dozen times, but then started finding excuses not to go.

I think AA is a wonderful organisation. It has saved millions of lives around the globe and some of my friends can't live without it. I guess one of my problems with it was that I wasn't going there for the reasons I should have been going – for instance, because my drinking was impacting on other people and on my children. I just wanted to cure my depression, so I was very much in denial of my alcoholism and hadn't yet hit my rock bottom. But perhaps my main problem with it was that I never believed that a higher power would help me to stop drinking, which is a tenet of the AA programme. I always say willpower stopped me drinking, and I guess it was nice to have some support.

I gave up for about eighteen months, thinking that sobriety would bring me happiness and contentment. I kept wanting a miracle to happen; I kept waiting to suddenly feel amazing. In the evenings, I stayed at home painting kitchen chairs and doing other wholesome activities, but happiness and contentment remained elusive.

It didn't occur to me that I needed to try to mend the problems that were making me drink in the way I drank, including my marriage. I think Tim and I realised a long time before we separated that our marriage had gone wrong, but were both reluctant to admit it. Neither of us was in a good place and alcohol was very much a part of our lives, our social lives and our friends' lives. Our house was party central: Matthew and his pals were starting a band, and there were teenagers in and out at all hours. It was a crazy house and therefore it was very hard to be sober, especially as everyone around me was still drinking.

I don't know whether people took my sobriety seriously. I don't think I even took it seriously. I was sober, but I never felt like a sober person. Something in the back of my mind knew it wasn't permanent, even though my unwelcome visitor was mainly absent and I became convinced that not drinking was the key to keeping him at bay.

Then I hit an episode of black depression and my world fell apart. As the visitor arrived, I realised with utter dismay that I wasn't cured. It was devastating. I had to resign myself to the fact that my depressive illness was a lifelong condition. I wasn't going to get better.

I battled on, even though I desperately wanted to go out drinking with my friends and be part of things again. I was very unhappy. It wasn't just my marriage – there were many issues in my life that weren't right, and so I found it difficult to appreciate the wonderful side of sobriety that I enjoy now.

After finishing work on *Down To Earth* I had been cast as the inept French teacher, Steph Haydock, in the BBC TV series *Waterloo Road*, about life in a Rochdale comprehensive school. One night in the summer of 2006, Chris Geere and Philip Martin Brown, my two best friends at the show, said they were going to a barbecue later on. The way they were talking about it was very seductive. It was a beautiful summer's evening and they were using all the buzzwords that advertisers use to make alcohol sound alluring. 'Delicious, refreshing, cold beers ... chilled champagne ... cheeky glass of Beaujolais ... Sauvignon on ice ...'

That was the day I made the decision to 'step off the wagon', a phrase I invented to make it sound like a sexy and controlled move. I didn't want people to think I'd 'fallen off the wagon', because when I hear that expression I think of someone staring at a drink, desperate to down it, then picking it up, unable to resist, and knocking it back.

I wanted 'stepping off the wagon' to make me a special person. 'I think I've got my drinking under control now,' I told people. 'And now that I know that it's not what's causing my depression, I'll just enjoy the odd little drink with friends of a Friday evening.'

Within a fortnight of starting drinking again I was as bad as I had been before, and worse.

I've never met a problem drinker who was able to cut down on their drinking for long. I've met people who have convinced themselves that, by giving up for a short time, they're all right now, but I don't think they are. It doesn't matter what I think, though. It's their business – I'm not the drink police. However, when asked for advice, I always want to say, 'If you have a bad relationship with alcohol, stop drinking if you can. Don't just cut down, because it's unlikely to make things any better.'

'Oh, but I don't have a problem. I don't drink in the week. I just drink at weekends,' people say, and even though they collapse and have blackouts, or get into fights or abuse their family, they have this misconception that their drinking isn't a problem because they lay off it during the week. But they do have a drink problem.

Giving up alcohol doesn't cure clinical depression, but it stops it being compounded. When you suffer from any mental health issue, drinking just makes you ten times worse. I, more than anybody, understand that having a drink has a brief numbing effect, but you've got to get past that because, by numbing the pain for a short time, you're lengthening the time it will stay with you. Alcohol is a depressant, not a stimulant, and you only have to look at your friends crying because they've had gin to know it. Everybody cries after gin, even if it's only, 'I love you so much, you don't realise how much . . .'

I generally don't think about drinking now; there have been a couple of times when an episode of depression has tested my sobriety, but never so much that I have seriously considered having a drink. I draw strength in knowing that if I drank, instead of staying three days the unwelcome visitor might well linger for three weeks. Then I would be right back in the vicious circle of drinking to numb the pain and making it worse. That's why the best thing anyone with any kind of mental health issue can do for themselves is take alcohol out of their life. It will not cure your illness, but it will have a hugely advantageous effect on how you manage your illness.

Although I started drinking again, I stopped thinking that my depression wasn't ever going to come back. I had to accept that it was something that I just had, like people have diabetes, and that it wasn't going to go away, that it was something I had to manage. Obviously it took me a long time to learn how to manage it, because I was managing it with self-medication, but that acceptance helped me to move forward nonetheless.

PART 4

Positive Steps

I

The first time I gave up drinking, the unwelcome visitor stayed away longer than usual: for more than six months. Somehow though, when he reappeared I forgot this, maybe because I was so disappointed to see him again. I had been under the illusion that he wouldn't return, so when he did, it was a real struggle to keep going and keep battling what I had now realised was a lifelong illness. It was inevitable that I would start self-medicating again.

I had never stopped searching for an effective treatment for my depression. When I became poorly again in 2007, despite being sober, I felt so bad that I went to The Priory, a private mental health care hospital in Altrincham, and asked to see a psychiatrist.

'Something happens to me physically and it affects my brain almost immediately,' I told the psychiatrist when I saw him.

I explained that my illness could come on within thirty seconds, in a whoosh, from my toes up.

He looked puzzled. 'What do you mean? Can you describe it in a little more detail?' He spoke with a mid-European accent that made him sound like a cross between Inspector Clouseau and Sigmund Freud.

'Well, I can be okay and then it comes out of nowhere, or I can bring it on myself, with the fear of the fear of it,' I said. 'It often happens at an important moment – for instance, if I'm going onstage, or on a live TV show like *Loose Women*, or just before my fortieth birthday party, I think, "Wouldn't it be awful if . . . Oh God, wouldn't it be awful if I got my thing?" and then I feel hot, the blackness goes up me like a whoosh, and it's on me.'

'I see,' he said, looking thoughtful. 'You describe "the whoosh". What I think you have is temporal lobe epilepsy.'

'What's that?' I asked.

'Well, it's very serious, because you can't drive a car in case you have a seizure. They'll take away your licence,' he said.

'Would it cause depression?'

'Yes, it would certainly cause it.'

'Can we look at my hormones, too, please?' I asked him. 'Because I was fine until I had a baby and I've always assumed that the origin of my depression is hormonal.'

He shook his head vigorously. 'No, it's not the hormones. No, no, no!'

'But why would this illness affect so many women when they have a baby?'

'There is nothing to prove the hormones,' he insisted. 'All the women say the hormones. But everybody has the hormones.'

I wasn't convinced, but I was desperate to be given an alternative diagnosis if it meant that I had something treatable, or even curable. I longed for someone to say, 'You've been mistreated for so many years! You don't need antidepressants – you've got temporal lobe epilepsy, and here's the tablet to make you better. You can never drive a car again, but it doesn't matter, because you're cured. You will never have your illness again.'

Although I have since discovered that temporal lobe epilepsy is a horrendous condition and I wouldn't wish it on my worst enemy, I was actually dismayed when the results of my brain scan and blood tests came back negative. I just wanted a diagnosis.

I consulted other doctors, but they shrugged and said, 'We haven't a clue how to deal with this.'

I was no closer to finding answers. And so the greyness continued.

For this reason, I have contradictory memories of the five years I spent on *Waterloo Road*. There were so many good things about the show: it was filmed in Rochdale so I was able to be based at home while we were filming; and I had a fantastic role in Steph Haydock. Steph was a secondary character when I first went into the show, but I made her my own and the writers loved writing for her because she was just fabulous. Before long, she became a leading light of the series.

The cast were amazing people and remain friends to this day. There was a whole bunch of ages, with actors from age eleven right the way up to me and Philip Martin Brown, a wonderful actor, who played Grantly Budgen, my nemesis. It was a great show; it's rerunning now and seems to be as popular as ever. Many of the young actors from it have gone on to become Hollywood stars.

There were wonderful times at *Waterloo Road*, but I was also really struggling with my illness. For what seemed like months on end, I lived in a fog of survival, getting up in the morning in a greyness, working in a greyness and not talking to people about it.

By then, I was used to the good periods lasting much longer than the bad, so now that the bad was suddenly outweighing the good, I felt I was losing the battle with my depression. I realise now that the shift might have been related to the start of the menopause. At the time, I was terrified that the visitor was becoming a permanent fixture.

As I've said, sometimes grey depression is worse than black depression. When the visitor enters the house, wearing a black cloak, and shuts the door and stays, the depression can be so thick and dark that it forces you to stop, because there is no way that you can continue. But with grey depression, you can carry on, because the visitor doesn't come in. He hovers nearby or stays outside, knocking on the door, and although the incessant knock-knock-knocking can be very hard to live with, it doesn't force you to stop. You can work through it, and I did – I even won Best Actress for my role as Steph in *Waterloo Road* two years running at the *TV Quick* Awards, up against some cracking performers.

I've recognised the signs of grey depression in people's eyes when I've done talks on my illness and they have approached me to speak about it afterwards. I can usually tell when people are living in the greyness. If they've been through a traumatic event or, indeed, had a baby, they sometimes think it's natural to be feeling depressed. They think, 'Well, this is just how life is now.'

This is why mild depression is often harder to diagnose and treat than severe depression.

Waterloo Road was a bit like a soap opera: if you were a regular, the days were sometimes fourteen hours long and you packed a lot of scenes into each day. Often, I'd be picked up by my driver at six in the morning and wouldn't get back until seven or eight at night, sometimes later. Even then, I couldn't rest up at home because I had a small child to be present for, if he was still up. Sometimes I was so tired out from working and living in the grey that all I wanted to do was go to bed or have a drink, but Louis was my priority and I'd always try to focus on him before I collapsed into bed.

I had a couple of drivers who took me to and from the *Waterloo Road* set. On long-term jobs, you get to know your drivers so well that they become like hairdressers, in that you start to pour your heart out to them. My drivers knew all about my illness. The moment I got in the car, they knew what sort of day it was for me. The 'normal me', even at six o'clock in the morning, is quite lively and chatty. On the days when I wasn't well, it would be hard for me to say anything.

'Are you all right, Den? You're not today, are you?' they'd say.

I'd have a pillow in the car so that I could grab an extra half-hour's kip if I had the chance. On bad days I'd get in and lie down, not necessarily sleeping, but pretending to be, so that I didn't have to talk. The old 'I've got a tricky tummy' excuse would come out – and then, when I started drinking again, there were hangovers.

It didn't help that we were filming on a grim estate in the rainiest corner of the country. No matter whether we left my house in sunlight or snow, the sky always seemed to be dark and grey by the time we reached Kirkholt. One of my enduring memories is of standing outside with the smokers, in the doorway of a dilapidated school, puffing away in the sideways rain.

In the middle of all this fog, it was the actress Beverley Callard's fiftieth and she was having a do in a club in Manchester. I felt too poorly to go really, but it was my good friend's fiftieth and it was important to me to be there. I went on my own, knowing that I was bound to know lots of people. The unwelcome visitor followed behind, wearing grey; he was going everywhere with me at that time.

One of my best friends, Daran Little, was at the party, and I confided in him that I wasn't well. 'Yes, I can see it in your eyes,' he said. 'Are you okay?'

'I'm not, Daran. I'm losing the will,' I replied. 'I'm going through the motions, but I'm poorly.'

'What does your doctor say?' he asked.

'None of the doctors I've seen know how to treat it,' I said.

I had been researching treatments online and told Daran that I was planning to see a hormone specialist in Baltimore. 'I was a perfectly normal person until a human being formed inside me and I pushed that human being out of me,' I said. 'I'm sure hormones are the key.'

Daran frowned. 'Funnily enough, I've heard of a doctor in London who treats depression with hormones,' he said.

He told me that he had a good friend, another actress, who'd had great results with Professor John Studd, a doctor in Wimpole Street, W1. My heart would have leapt if I hadn't been feeling so low.

I always followed up recommendations people gave me; I snatched at them like a drowning man. So the next morning, standing in a corridor of the *Waterloo Road* school, I phoned Professor Studd's office and spoke to his secretary, Joan.

'My name is Denise Welch and I've been recommended to come and see Professor Studd,' I said, in a quivery, emotional voice. 'I'm suffering from depression and have done for many years, and I've heard that the professor treats depression that may have a hormonal origin.'

'When can you come?' Joan asked.

'Next week,' I said.

'Well, you get yourself down here to Wimpole Street and he will make you better,' Joan said.

It was a big statement: *He will make you better.* I'm not sure exactly why I believed her, but I took great solace in her words and kept repeating them to myself.

Professor Studd, when I first met him, was a giant of a man and as gruff and forthright as they come. I was feeling lucid that day and was more talkative than usual. As I was gabbling away about my mental health history, he said, 'Right, shut up, I've got the gist.'

'Wow, okay,' I said, unused to his particular style of bedside manner.

Within minutes, Professor Studd had taken out my Mirena contraceptive coil. 'I think you might be progesterone intolerant,' he said.

There was a massive machine in his office that could do blood tests on the spot and before long he discovered that my oestrogen levels were almost at zero. 'You are so deficient in oestrogen that I don't know how you've survived,' he said.

Just hearing those words brought me to tears. 'Why has it taken me twenty years for someone to say that the origin of my torture has been hormonal?' I asked him.

The lack of understanding about hormones in the medical profession is rooted in history, I think. Historically, women's health wasn't prioritised in the way that men's health was, and post-natal depression only happened to women. Since there are lots of women who don't get it, there was also an element of: 'Well, look at Joyce: she was at a disco three nights after she gave birth!' or, as my GP in London said, 'I had five children, dear, and I just didn't have time to get depressed.'

Since, in the eyes of society, we were destined for the scrapheap once we couldn't bear children any more, there was never going to be any investment in our mental health. Until hormone replacement therapy (HRT) was developed to counteract the changes that occur during menopause, when you stopped menstruating – unless you were lucky – you went mad, no one cared and your husband went off and had an affair because you were old and constantly angry.

As well as treating women for post-natal and prenatal depression, Professor Studd had patients suffering with premenstrual syndrome (PMS). Like post-natal depression, PMS can be a severe illness. Our hormones are so powerful that women with severe PMS can go for two weeks out of every month from being normal, caring, nurturing wives and mothers to having murderous impulses and trying to stab their husbands. It's horrible for everybody. For years all that doctors prescribed was tranquillisers, which just turn people into zombies.

Professor Studd treated me with hormone replacement therapy – lots of oestrogen, a little progesterone and some testosterone to boost my sex drive – and I felt better within about a week. It made an incredible difference. It was like a miracle. It didn't cure me of my illness and I went on to have episodes of depression again, but it helped me enormously in my day-to-day survival and I'll be forever grateful. It was fantastic to feel 'normal' again. I wasn't skipping through the tulips, unless something happened to inspire me to skip through the tulips, but I felt able to approach my working day as any other actress would.

As I write this book, *Waterloo Road* is streaming on iPlayer. Lincoln had never seen it and so I hand-picked a few episodes for him recently and we sat and watched them together. 'I wasn't well that day,' I'd say, whenever we came to a scene where I remembered having depression. What was comforting was that he couldn't detect a difference between my performance when I was ill and when I was well. Only I could tell.

Acceptance of this illness is key to a quicker recovery and a better life between episodes, but unfortunately I wasn't yet ready to stop drinking, which compounded my depression. Staying off alcohol isn't easy in a culture that actively encourages people to consume it. When on top of having depression you're unhappy in your marriage and working all hours, it's particularly hard to resist. I felt I didn't have the strength to keep going without it.

I probably used the visitor's return as an excuse to drink again. 'It hasn't stopped my depression; where's the red wine?'

But it wasn't just my illness; I can't say that I was drinking just to self-medicate. *Waterloo Road* was party central and I was working with a lot of people who enjoyed a drink. We were all doing it.

Of course, a normal person comes into work after a big night, saying, 'Oh God, I feel terrible, give me a fry-up!'

They've still got their sense of humour and can laugh through the pain of the hangover; it's purely physical for them.

But hard drinking would take me to another level, to a horrible place. And yet I would do it again and again.

When I was ill, the instant respite from the alcohol helped me. When I was unhappy, it relieved my emotional pain. When I was hungover and depressed, it put me back on an even keel. Alcohol was a great short-term fix, but it solved nothing in the long term. It just made everything worse.

The ITV daytime talk show *Loose Women* has been a part of my life for a long time now, and over the years it has given me a fabulous platform to talk about mental health and get the message out. I began making regular appearances on the show in 2002, when it was a much smaller production and filmed in Manchester. Then it relocated to Norwich and we had to re-audition for our roles. The auditions lasted a couple of days and all sorts of famous people came along, from journalists and commentators to actors, presenters and models. It was a complete potpourri of women, all vying for the *Loose Women* slots. I remember being there with Coleen Nolan, thinking, 'What if we don't get it again?'

Eventually, I was offered the Friday slot from Norwich, with Fiona Phillips anchoring and me, Jaci Stephen and the wonderful Alison Hammond on the panel. I loved everything about taking part in the show, apart from getting there, which was a nightmare for me: I was still terrified of flying and the only way to reach Norwich without doing a six-hour drive was to fly.

Every week, I had this 40-minute white-knuckle ride in a tiny plane with just a curtain between me and the pilot. The pilot used to have to talk me through the journey because I was so scared. He'd turn to me and say, 'I'm putting the wheels down now, Denise, so there's going to be a bump.'

'Okay,' I'd whisper through clenched teeth, going grey.

It was worth it, though, because *Loose Women* was always

such good fun. I'm a real girl's girl – or a woman's woman – and I hate it when people try to imply that there has to be lots of backbiting and bitching on a show like *Loose Women*, when there isn't.

All was going well until my agent rang me one day and said, 'Just to let you know, they won't be getting in touch with you about your travel tomorrow. They're doing something different and don't need you to be there.'

'What do you mean?' I asked, sensing that she was choosing her words delicately.

'They're not being very clear. Just sit tight for this one and then we'll establish what's happening.'

I instantly felt panicked. It was the not knowing that made it so bad. My stomach started churning, my heart began racing and my mouth went dry. The next day, when I turned on the television to watch the show, the actress Rebecca Wheatley was sitting in my seat. I had been replaced, with no phone call, no letter, nothing. It was horrible. I'm old and ugly enough to deal with things if someone gives me an explanation – even if I don't agree with that explanation – but somebody didn't like me and nobody bothered to explain.

I had a pretty miserable time of it, but producers change, and whoever came in next wanted me back. I rejoined the show after it went to London in 2004 and was a regular panellist for the next nine years, until 2013, when I stepped back for a while.

After that early blip, *Loose Women* supported me and made me feel like a valued member of the team through some very dark times in my life. I was a bit of a car wreck at times because, although I had finally got the hormone replacement treatment I had needed for so long, I was still very unhappy. What made it worse was that I didn't realise just how unhappy I was.

Loose Women was there for me through it all and tried to embrace the party-animal, 'Drunk Spice' identity that I carved out on the show. I was the one who said, 'So what if you're in your late forties and you're out until 4 a.m.? Come on, everybody!' and, 'Infidelity isn't the worst thing that can happen in a marriage! What, Jackie Brambles? You would finish with Dave if he snogged someone else? How pathetic! I'm "Drunk Spice", I'm out there!'

Honestly, I would hate to see the playback of those shows. I'm in a different place now; I'm a different person. If Lincoln kissed someone else, it would be the end of my life, metaphorically, which shows how much I have changed. I pretended to be this funster who didn't care about being outrageous, but I was really trying to justify being someone I didn't like.

Although my depressive episodes were fewer and farther between now that I was on HRT, they hadn't gone away. When I was ill, people often asked, 'What do you think brought this episode on?' I didn't drink every day; often there was no reason at all for the visitor to appear. At times, it just felt like I was being stalked by an insane assassin.

In 2010, at the height of the American romcom drama *Sex and the City*'s popularity, myself, Lisa Maxwell, Sherrie Hewson and Carol McGiffin were given the chance to go to New York to make a '*Loose Women* on location' DVD. What could be more fabulous than going away to film in New York with your pals? Off we went with our production team: we flew business class and stayed in an amazing hotel. Since I had always dreamt of filming in America, I felt as if I was ticking all the boxes of exciting things to do. We had five days in Manhattan and our schedule was packed with all kinds of great activities.

On our second night we sat out on the roof terrace of our hotel, having drinks, looking over Manhattan. 'Oh my goodness, this is amazing!' I thought. It was like being in a movie.

We had an early start the next morning – each of us had a make-up artist coming to our room at 7 a.m. – so, after two vodka and tonics, I went to bed. Before I fell asleep, I looked out of my window at the row of brownstone houses across the street from our hotel. My heart leapt with excitement. 'Wow, I'm in New York!'

But my first thought when I woke up in the morning was, 'Oh no, he's here.' I got up and paced around my hotel room. 'You're not coming!' I told the unwelcome visitor. 'Absolutely not!'

By the time the make-up artist arrived, I could hardly speak.

It was awful. There was nothing I could do. I couldn't ring down and say, 'I don't feel well. I can't work today.'

Although I say now that I would be kinder to myself these days, four of us had been hand-picked to go to New York and I was one of the four. So I got my make-up on and went to meet the others in the lobby.

We were filming in Carnegie Deli, the famous delicatessen that featured in almost every New York movie made before it closed down in 2016, the one with photographs of Mafia figures covering the walls. It was known for selling the tallest pastrami sandwiches in the city; but being ill, I had no appetite. Everything tasted like sandpaper and I couldn't eat a single morsel.

I tried to hide how I was feeling from the other girls, even though I knew they would understand. Everybody was up to high doh with excitement, enjoying this brilliant experience in New York City, and I didn't want to ruin it for them. It was bad enough that it was ruined for me.

As we got ready to film, I started to panic. 'I want to get out. I want to get out. I want to get out!'

One of my covers when I'm ill is to say I have cystitis, because if you say you have a girly condition in mixed company, no one questions it. 'I'm just off to the toilet. You know, got *cystitis* . . .' I whispered.

Then I was out on the street – breathing hard and walking around the block to try to distract myself – before I went back in and tried to appear normal again.

I don't remember much more of the trip, apart from going to Milk Studios for a photoshoot, where I was given a beautiful long dress to wear and stood in front of the cameras, trying to smile naturally.

The studios had put on an amazing spread for us and people kept saying, 'Are you not eating?'

'You know, I've got this *cystitis* . . . it's really given me a tummy ache. I'm fine, though. I've got enough reserves (patting my tummy) . . . and it won't do me any harm not to eat, just this once.'

Later on, I put on a red dress with a frilly collar to film a segment in 'my apartment'. I was supposed to welcome the girls, one by one, into my glorious apartment in New York, where we would have cocktails on 'my roof terrace'.

'You all right, babes?' McGiff asked me.

'I'm not, Carol,' I said.

'Oh, babes,' she said.

It's funny with McGiff, because she's never really understood clinical depression, but she never, ever disputed that I had something really bad. She was always very supportive.

Next, I had to interview Lisa, Sherrie and Carol, and all the while I could feel my mouth stiffening. Nobody would have known, watching it on the video, but as we were chatting away, I was thinking, 'Look at them! They're all fine. They're just sitting on this rooftop enjoying the twinkly lights of New York, feeling normal. Nobody knows what I'm going through.'

That night when I went to bed, I hoped that the visitor would be gone when I woke up the next morning. But he was there from the moment I opened my eyes.

The day before we left, we were scheduled to go out into Times Square to ask members of the public jokey questions, like, 'Have you ever heard of a British show called *Loose Women*?'

It was the sort of thing I would normally have had a lot of fun with, but I was feeling so poorly that I could barely speak. 'I can't,' I told Karl, our producer.

'All right,' he said. 'The others can do your bit.'

Afterwards, Lisa Maxwell and I did a mad dash to Toys"R"Us to get presents for people, and I started to feel even worse. In a thick fog, I crouched down in a corner of this huge toy store and rang Tim. My depression was so bad that I just needed to hear someone say, 'You're all right. You've only got one more day. You're coming home tomorrow. Just get through it. If you can't do anything, just go to bed. Nobody will die.'

Before we left, we visited Ground Zero, where I felt absolutely nothing, because I was so depressed. What a horrible illness it is, to rob you of the emotion you want to feel at Ground Zero.

When we checked out of our hotel at the end of the trip, I could feel my depression lifting, perhaps because I was relieved that I didn't have to work through it any more. As we got on the plane and I watched McGiff go straight to the business-class bar, I laughed genuinely for the first time in days. Carol went on to get so drunk that it was a struggle to get her back to her seat in time for landing. Once seated, she fell asleep and when she woke up she thought we were back in New York!

There were a few years during my late forties and early fifties when all I was doing was chasing my tail with my illness, just trying to get through. It was one big round of trying to self-medicate being ill and being unhappy; I hit the bottle and it was all a bit of a blur. The feeling of doing anything you can to stop the pain can, unfortunately, set up an extremely destructive pattern in your life. I was a lost soul and I went down a very dark rabbit hole.

I don't blame anybody or anything for my behaviour. But there were reasons why my life became so dark. One reason was that my marriage was not working and neither of us wanted to admit to it. Another was that I was being hacked by the newspapers. The repercussions of being hacked took me to the depths of horror; I spent a period of several years not trusting anybody, not even my closest friends. It was soul-destroying.

Who could ever have imagined the extent of the phone hacking that we now know went on? Thousands of lives have been blighted by it. I know people who fell out with their families because they thought their close relatives were selling stories on them. After all, they reasoned, who else knew they were in Glasgow, or pregnant, apart from the one family member they had confided in? They had no idea that the newspapers were listening in to every last detail. Sadly, when the truth came to light, often their families couldn't forgive their lack of trust in them.

Trust first became an issue for me while I was working at *Coronation Street*. The V&A Hotel in Manchester was a big party destination and the press always seemed to find out who was there, with whom, doing what. Years later, we found out that one of the V&A concierges was on the payroll of a tabloid newspaper, which happened in many major hotels, apparently – and still does. It was sad, because this was someone we had all befriended and trusted, but he was completely two-faced and selling us down the river. Unfortunately, he was so devious that he escaped all suspicion and instead I thought that a couple of my friends might be selling stories – and once that seed was planted, it grew.

During my hacking case against the *Mirror*, which was settled out of court in 2016, I spent five hours in Putney police station sifting through police evidence of what had been uncovered. To my horror, I found myself looking at my private life and realising that none of it had been private. I discovered that when I was having an affair with Steve Murray, the carpenter on the set of *Down To Earth*, the press rented the flat above the estate agents opposite his house in Marlow, Buckinghamshire, to spy on us. For two weeks! I also found out that the papers had followed Steve to Cuba on his holidays to try to trick him into selling a story, and there was information on Myra, the attractive journalist who had 'befriended' me in the toilets of the Knightsbridge wine bar and later sold a story on me.

This is little old me! It's not like I'm some major Hollywood star. Can you imagine what the royal family go through? It's unbelievable how cut-throat the papers are.

Before all the hacking was exposed – in that age of innocence – how was I to know that two guys had put a bug in my room at the St George's Hotel in Regent Street? So, when a cast member saw Steve Murray come out of my hotel bedroom, and then the press found out, it wasn't a wild leap of fancy to assume that the cast member had told someone about it. I didn't think he had rung the city desk at the *Mirror* and reported seeing the set carpenter coming out of my bedroom, but perhaps he'd gone back to work and said, 'You won't believe who I just saw . . .' and that piece of general gossip had got to the papers.

What else was I going to think? I had no reason to suspect that there was a listening device in my hotel room – that was the stuff of spy films.

I was in a constant state of paranoia during this time. I'm not looking for sympathy – I was being unfaithful, because I was unhappy in my marriage – but the hacking definitely played a part in my subsequent mental health downfall. It led to not trusting people I loved, because every time I met a friend for a drink, or poured out my heart on the phone, the press seemed to know about it. When I voiced my suspicions, my friends furiously denied doing anything wrong; they begged me to believe them, but the doubt remained. These were people I had known for twenty or thirty years, so it really shook me. My old friend, Lester, for instance: I had been with Lester the night the press took pap pictures of me that were later used in the *Mirror* after I'd been entrapped by Myra, the cousin of the fake sheik, Mazir Mahmoud; I thought that maybe Lester had let something slip to his boyfriend who had talked to the press, and even though he swore he hadn't, I couldn't be sure. But if I couldn't trust Lester, then who could I trust? My life seemed to get messier by the day, which played into my depression, and I felt I had no one to turn to.

The way my drinking was documented in the media over the years must have made people wonder how I held down a job and never got fired, let alone raised my two children. At times, it must have looked like I was out every night, staggering around the streets of London, or Manchester, or wherever I happened to be. I'm sure my career took a hit because of it. Every photo of me taken outside an event or a club would be angled to make me look plastered – even when I hadn't had a sip of alcohol. The papers simply decided what the story was and shaped their photos and text around it. Hacking my phone gave them the chance to pap me every time I went out. There were photographers lurking around unexpected corners and a lot of concocted articles about my life spiralling out of control, with accompanying pap shots. It was horrible. I'm not saying that I didn't do bad things and put myself in the firing line, but if journalists are listening to your calls, you're such an easy target. When they know who you're talking to and where you're going – and as a result you lose trust in everybody in your life – it's going to break you. I was incredibly vulnerable, and it broke me.

My life was unravelling and I couldn't see a way out. I wasn't alone in turning to drink to deal with family problems, work difficulties and depression – it's something that millions of people around the world do every day – but it was making things worse and I didn't have the strength to stop it. Things were nowhere near as bad as the press made them look, though. I am not proud of the fact that sometimes I partied all night and went straight to work in the morning, but I still managed to be an award-winning actress and presenter. I've always turned up to work on time, always done a good job and been professional and fun to work with. Anybody who knows me knows that I was never staggering around.

However, being hacked was enough to make you question your sanity and plunge you down to rock bottom, even if you didn't have clinical depression.

III

People have a false conception of what it means to have an alcohol problem. It doesn't always mean hiding bottles of gin, drinking in the morning, knocking back vodka in the car and all the things that some alcoholics do. However I was portrayed in the media, I was never a mother who opened the cleaning cupboard at nine o'clock in the morning and reached to the back to find a hidden bottle of vodka that I could pour into my coffee. I wasn't that person, just as I wasn't somebody who drank every single evening. My problem was being unable to admit to myself that I didn't have an off-button. 'I won't do what I did the other night,' I'd say, as I poured myself a large glass of red wine. 'I'm just going to have a couple and go to bed.'

Then the same thing would happen all over again: I'd drink too much and wake up with a hangover and depression, berating myself; I'd try to get through the day without making the depression any worse; I'd drink again in the evening just to feel okay. It just went on and on and on. I spent years of my life not living, but getting through the day until I could have a drink, go to sleep or go and lie in a room on my own and deal with what was going on in my head.

Being a regular on *Loose Women* from 2004 to 2013 meant that I spent a lot of time in London, and it often felt as if I was living a separate life to Tim. We were trying to keep our marriage together at home, but with both of us being away working, we were a bit like those people who have one family in London and another hidden away in the heart of the countryside.

We felt we were doing the right thing by staying married, but in hindsight we weren't – not for us and not for the children. We were aware that we didn't love each other like we should. We had moved on in our minds, but were too terrified to physically move on, and I felt very dependent on Tim to get me through my depressive episodes. We wanted to keep the family together, so we tried to live our own lives within the confines of pretending that our marriage was okay.

Like many couples, we concealed what was going on beneath the surface by drinking together, and drinking causes arguments. It was so destructive, for us and everybody around us. We tried not to argue in front of the children, but the sad fact is that kids whose parents are self-medicating and whose marriages are breaking down see and hear too much. It's something that's going on in homes all over the world, among people from every type of background. The alcohol consumes their rows and fuels their anger and nastiness.

The day after an argument, when people say, 'I didn't mean that,' it's usually not true. People don't say things they don't mean; they just say things they don't mean to say out loud. Before they know it, there's no coming back from it, because the words have been said. They can't put the genie back in the bottle.

Tim and I said a lot of things we didn't mean to say, and yet I didn't think that splitting up was an option. 'I'm married to him and he's the boys' dad. I can't leave,' I thought.

We neither of us wanted to admit it was over, because we had a dependency on each other. Whether or not we were making each other happy became irrelevant. We had been together for twenty-four years and we had two children. We were also a 'show-business couple', so it felt as if there was a lot resting on Tim and Denise being together. The stories I told on *Loose Women* were often about Tim, and the reason they were so hilarious was because Tim was a famous and respected actor. People viewed us affectionately as 'naughty Denise' and 'long-suffering Tim', which was funny until the affection turned to criticism.

Down in London, I let loose the party animal in me. I had lots of people hanging on my coat-tails. 'Here she is!' would go up the cry when I arrived in a bar. 'We'll go to all the clubs and parties now she's here! She'll get us in!'

I thought that if I was giving people a good time, I must be a good person and it was fine to go on doing it. But of course, after a night of partying and madness, they'd go home and sleep and lie in the next day and wake up feeling a bit groggy, go out for a fry-up and, Bob's your uncle, everything would be all right. Meanwhile, I'd be plunged into this blackness and have to go to work. It's nobody's fault but my own, but I didn't know how to stop.

In the midst of all this came the crazy night in February 2011 when I met Lincoln. It's the only thing I have to thank my drinking for, actually. It all began when I was turned away from a BRITs after-party at the Savoy Hotel, because I arrived with twenty people. I had gone out with a couple of friends and ended up with twenty! By this time, the newspapers had stopped hacking my phone, and yet the photographers seemed to be expecting me; I was papped being turned away at the hotel entrance.

I had no desire to go to the BRITs (the irony being that my son is now a three-time BRITs winner!) but I was invited to the after-party by a friend. Over the course of the evening I had gathered my tribe, like the Pied Piper of Soho, and we all trooped merrily down from Soho House to this party.

'You can't come in,' the doorman said.

'What do you mean, I can't come in?' I said, aghast. 'I'm on the guest list!'

'Yes, you're on the guest list, Denise, but not the twenty people you've brought with you!'

'Bollocks to you!' I threw my arms in the air, and was papped.

The hangers-on drifted away and about eight of us decided to go on somewhere. Apparently we gatecrashed Tinie Tempah's party. 'Don't you remember, Mum?' Matthew asked me a few months ago. 'You and your bunch of pals walked into Tinie Tempah's party and George said, "There's your mother," and we exited out the other door.'

I have no recollection of it. Why would I be at Tinie Tempah's party? I don't know.

At that point, though, I was having fun, even though I don't remember it now. 'Where to next?' I asked, hailing a taxi.

'Jet Black!' someone said.

Jet Black was a club that didn't open until 2 a.m. and didn't close until 6 a.m. Once we got there, according to my friends, I disappeared, and to this day nobody knows where I went. I just remember coming through a door and finding that all of my friends had gone. I was fuming! In my mind, I had been away five minutes, but they all swear that I was gone for an hour. Please tell me where I was, because I don't know!

The club was almost empty by then. My friend Noel Watson came over with a smartly dressed man. 'Hi Den, this is my friend Lincoln, from Stringfellows,' he said.

(He was listed under 'Lincoln from Stringfellows' on my phone until long after we were married!)

Who would have thought that a man working in a job in the lap-dance world, out at a nightclub, also with alcohol issues, who I met at three o'clock in the morning, would become the love of my life ten years on? It's unbelievable, but that's what happened. That meeting at three in the morning was the catalyst that changed my life for ever.

Lincoln and I instantly got on and exchanged numbers when I left Jet Black, shortly afterwards. After that, we rang each other sometimes and saw each other now and again.

Then, just as we were starting to become closer, the press found out. Of course!

'But how did they find out?' I wondered.

We would meet for a drink at a hotel off the beaten track, leave by the back entrance and get papped the moment we stepped outside. Unaware that someone in my close circle was leaking stories about me, I would have been a fool not to suspect Lincoln of tipping off the papers that we were there.

'Who is this Lincoln from Stringfellows?' my friends said. 'Why are you trusting him?'

'I would never, ever talk to the papers about you,' Lincoln swore to me, and I believed him, despite how it looked. I felt drawn to him. I wanted to be with him.

Unbeknownst to the media, Tim and I had agreed to separate in early 2012. But yet again the press was accusing me of being 'an adulteress', because I was out on the town with a mystery man, leaving 'long-suffering Tim' at home.

I decided that I'd had enough. I was done with the way I was being treated and needed to take the power back from the press, who had completely invented their own narrative of my life. I spoke to the team at *Loose Women* about what was happening. 'Would you like to announce the separation on live television?' they suggested.

I spoke to Tim and the children and we agreed that I would do exactly that. It was heartbreaking and traumatic and upsetting to do, but I needed to say, 'I'm not cheating on my husband. Tim and I separated some time ago, but we just haven't chosen to share it with anybody until now.'

We had separated when I went into the *Big Brother* house six weeks earlier, and so taking part in *Celebrity Big Brother* had been a very lonely time for me. Nobody knew about the separation from Tim and nobody knew I was with Lincoln – and I couldn't talk about any of it to anybody.

When I came out of the house, having won *Celebrity Big Brother*, despite having a diabolical time, the press treated me very badly. It was all over the papers that I was having an affair and my friends told me that Lincoln had been selling stories about me. But it wasn't Lincoln. Years later, someone who worked with me admitted that they had been the one selling stories about me, because they were resentful that I was breaking away from their influence. They threw me to the wolves and suddenly my life was in freefall, because everybody was saying I was a horrible person for being unfaithful to Tim.

Throughout it all, Lincoln was there for me and our relationship was blossoming. But we had a big problem. I was self-medicating like crazy, partly because of all the negative press about me, and Lincoln was also drinking too much. Alcohol was stopping us from moving forward. Unfortunately, it's something I often see: two people have a really good relationship, but alcohol is messing it up.

I gave Lincoln an ultimatum. 'I don't want to be with the person you are when you drink,' I said.

I took the higher ground, because I felt I didn't have as much of a problem as he did. I felt that I wasn't mean and nasty when I drank, but actually I *was* mean and nasty to the people who cared about me and had concerns about me. If any of my loved ones tried to suggest my drinking was out of control, I lashed out. The idea of sobriety filled me with dread.

'If you love me, you'll stop drinking,' I said.

Lincoln stopped drinking for good that day in February 2012. I didn't give up but decided to cut down. I was starting an important job – a touring production of the play *Steel Magnolias* – and thought I would be able to limit my drinking while I was doing it.

By the time I went on tour, Lincoln had left Stringfellows and was working on private parties and PR projects, so he was driving me around and doing his work on the hop.

One morning, in Brighton, he said, 'You were horrible to me last night.'

'No, I wasn't,' I said.

I had woken up wondering why I felt hungover, but I didn't tell him that. 'I only had two glasses of wine,' I added.

'You think you only had a couple,' he said, 'but you had a couple in your dressing room after the play. Then we went to the pub with your friends and you had a couple. Then I drove you back and you had a couple. So you've had a bottle and a half of wine. I'm not monitoring what you drink, but I kind of am.'

'Oh, don't be so ridiculous,' I said.

'You were needling me, trying to spoil for a fight,' he told me.

'I wouldn't do that!' I protested.

The play moved on to Richmond, which was the nearest we were going to the West End, and the other girls in the show and I decided to invite our famous friends to come and see it, so that we could create a bit of a buzz for the rest of the tour. It was 18 April 2012 and a potpourri of people off the telly came along, from Derek Jacobi to Nanny Pat from *The Only Way is Essex*.

'Darling, there are going to be paps there tonight,' Lincoln said, as we were getting ready to go to the theatre. 'So if you start to get drunk, I'll tell you.'

'I won't get drunk,' I said. 'I've got two shows tomorrow.'

Fast-forward to Lincoln saying, 'Darling, I'm not lecturing you, but you are getting drunk. I know the friend you just snogged was gay, but the paps are taking pictures of you through the window.'

'Don't you tell me what to do!' I snapped.

'I'm just looking out for you,' he said.

I don't remember anything after that. I woke up in Lincoln's flat in Kensington the next morning to find the bathroom door had been broken, although I didn't know how. There was stuff flung on the floor. I had no idea why.

I soon found out. Although I couldn't remember a thing about it, Lincoln had videoed me furiously arguing with him and banging doors when we had got home. I was defensive at first and wouldn't listen to the recording when he started playing it back. 'I'm not the only person who's got drunk on a night out!' I said.

He showed me a copy of that day's newspaper with a photo of me leaning over the bonnet of a car, drunkenly pointing at him. There was nothing more I could say in my defence.

I had two shows to do that day. I don't know how I got through them, but I did. I went in and turned in two fantastic performances, and nobody in the audience would have known. But I knew how desperately poorly I felt, physically and mentally.

Lincoln picked me up at the end of the show that night. When I got in the car, he said, 'I don't want you to say a word. I just want you to listen.'

He talked to me non-stop from Richmond to Kensington, which was a journey of about half an hour. He talked about how deep his love was for me and what a wonderful person he thought I was, but how, now that he was sober and really trying hard with it, it was going to be impossible to move forward with someone who was drinking as much as I was.

'Would you prefer me to walk away?' he asked.

I shook my head.

He didn't ask me to stop drinking. He said, 'I've decided that if we go out, after you've had a couple of glasses of wine, I'm going to leave.'

I thought back to a previous relationship I'd been in and remembered the feeling of dread I'd had whenever I heard the key in the lock, because the man in question was so change-able that I never knew who was going to walk through the door.

'I'm not putting the man I love through that,' I thought. 'I don't want him not knowing which girlfriend is going to walk in – sober girlfriend, tiddly girlfriend or the I-want-an-argument-girlfriend.'

'I want to stop and I'm going to stop,' I said.

I haven't had a drink since that night.

It took meeting Lincoln for me to realise that if I gave up drinking and worked at it, I could have a different, much better life – not just for me, but for everybody else. Giving up alcohol in no way cures depression, but it stops compounding it and puts an end to your self-hatred and lack of self-esteem. It allows you to build up your sense of worth again and survive your illness, because you know that you are doing everything in your power to keep the visitor away. It makes your family happy; the people you love can live their lives free of worry about you and your safety. Because it's not what you're going to say or do to embarrass them that matters to them, it's your well-being, so it gives them – and you – a sense of peace.

All of these things limit the length of time that your depression stays – and when it comes, you don't bash yourself, thinking, 'Oh, if I hadn't drunk, the visitor wouldn't be here.'

You know that your depression is there because your body chemistry has changed, and you have done nothing that might have brought it on.

I just wish that I'd given up drinking sooner, but there's no point in thinking about it. I didn't have the strength. I wasn't in the right place. Tim and I were enabling each other. When I gave up the first time, he went on drinking, which made it more difficult. I'm not blaming Tim. I didn't give him an ultimatum. Anyway, my marriage wasn't in a good place, so the temptation was to drink again. But when it came to my relationship with Lincoln, I knew that it couldn't work with him being sober and me drinking. I was so in love with him that I couldn't allow our destructive addictions to ruin something wonderful. Alcohol seemed to keep things going with Tim, but with Lincoln it ruined things.

The love we had and my desire to change propelled us towards a new life. We had already come through so much together as a couple, with people lying about us, selling stories on us, our addictions, my depression, all of those things – was I going to let alcohol ruin this relationship? I chose not to.

Giving up drinking is the thing I'm most proud of, apart from my children. When I give a talk about my illness now, I know I couldn't stand up with the same certainty, confidence and knowledge if I were drinking. It gives me the ability to help other people, just by talking about my story. That's why I'm opening myself up and leaving myself vulnerable again by doing this book – because I feel it's my duty in life to do what I can to help people survive depression. I can't tell them how to survive it. I can only tell them what I do to survive it.

When we stopped drinking, Lincoln came up with the idea that we would be each other's anchors. We made a commitment to each other and to ourselves that, if anything were to happen to the other person, we would not go down that road again. I know that if I started drinking again, I would be betraying my love for Lincoln as well as for myself. For some people AA is their anchor, for others it's the risk of losing their children or partner.

People say, 'It was easy for you, because you had a partner,' and I can't deny that it was easier.

But I wish that my anchor had been something else before it was Lincoln. I've since gone on to find other anchors. Also anchoring me is knowing how my sobriety has transformed the lives of my children and changed the trajectory of their lives. As I sit here with Matthew being in one of the biggest bands in the world and Louis making his name as an actor, I believe that none of it would be possible if I were still drinking.

Of course, keeping the unwelcome visitor away is yet another anchor.

It was hard to give up – very, very hard – but I was madly in love with Lincoln, and things instantly change for the better if you are in a good place when you take alcohol out of your life. It soon became clear what an amazing time we were going to have together. Alcohol causes arguments and we didn't argue now that we didn't drink. The change was so quick. We learned a lot about each other as a couple, just through being sober in the mornings. I immediately felt that we could achieve a massive amount together. Striving to do something along-side another person felt absolutely amazing.

A fortnight after I'd stopped drinking, I went home to my parents' house and told my mother that I'd stopped. Mum had been living with cancer for twenty years and, three years earlier, had been told that her cancer was terminal. Only, Mum's decline was so gradual that she never looked as if she was dying of cancer. She just looked a little delicate.

I nearly didn't go that day. I was at York on the tour with the play and I woke up poorly with my illness. 'I don't want to go, Linc,' I said. 'I just want to stay in bed. I've got the show to do tonight. Can we go tomorrow?'

Lincoln still hadn't met my parents. 'But I'm going to London for work tomorrow,' he said, unable to disguise the disappointment in his voice. 'We've promised your mum and she's expecting us . . . Can you just push yourself to go? We're only ninety minutes away. If you can, let's just try.'

When we got home, Mum was up in the bedroom. That day, when I looked at her, was the first time I saw a woman dying of cancer. I had a feeling that this was the beginning of the end, and it was.

Of course, normally, a situation as emotional as that would have sent me straight to the fridge for a bottle of wine. 'I can't drink,' I thought. 'I can't do that to my mum. I've told her that

I'm not going to drink. She has to know that I've moved forward before she dies.'

Lincoln was with me all the time. He didn't know my mum – he didn't really know me that well – and yet he was with me during that period and I so needed him there.

When I walked out of Mum's bedroom, it was the last time she was lucid. If I hadn't gone, I might not have seen my mum awake again. She died a fortnight later, on my birthday.

After Mum died, my sister, Debbie, said to me, 'I'm really proud that you didn't drink through this.'

My sister hadn't been proud of me for a long time. I had let a lot of people down. So it meant a lot to me that she said that.

'In Mum's memory, for my relationship and family, this is the path that I'm on now,' I thought.

After I saw Mum lucid for the last time, I felt my depression lifting and I'm glad to say that it didn't come back over the following weeks. It meant I could be present for Mum as I said goodbye to her. I could be there for my dad, as well, and for the rest of my family, so that we could all be together sharing the same emotion and the same experience. It meant I could be there at the funeral, and help organise everything. I couldn't have done any of those things if I was depressed. I would have gone through the motions, but it would have been horrendous. This is another example of the difference between clinical and circumstantial depression. My mother, who I loved more than anything, died, and the visitor stayed away.

I wish Mum had lived long enough to see me now: it's one of my greatest regrets and I really struggle with it sometimes. Mum used to worry about me so, so much. But it gives me solace that she lived to see me stop drinking and I know how pleased she would be that I turned things around, not just for me but for the whole family. Mum is one of the anchors that helps keep me sober.

IV

Ever since I went public with my sobriety, people have been coming up to me and saying, 'Can I have a quick word? I'd love to give up drinking but I'm not funny without a glass of wine in my hand. How do you do it?'

I know what they're thinking: 'Isn't life boring if you can't have a drink or two of an evening? How do you manage to have fun? And how do you cope if you can't switch off after a stressful day, or give yourself a bit of a lift when you're feeling down?'

Now, I don't ever want anyone to think I have all the answers, because I haven't. Yet I can safely say that in my experience, sobriety is great fun. It sounds boring but it's fun. On the flip side, drinking alcohol sounds like fun, but if your hangovers are accompanied by guilt, anxiety, self-loathing, nausea, horror, regret and depression, as mine sometimes were, it's the opposite of a good time.

It wasn't easy giving up. Getting through tough times, disappointments, daily stresses and worry about kids was tough without a drink to take the edge off. Thinking about my anchors stopped me picking up a glass of wine, though. It was so important for our children – including Lincoln's son, Lewis, who has health issues and can't drink alcohol – that neither Lincoln nor I were drinking.

Another big challenge I faced was to extricate myself from all those places and situations I associated with drink. I found it hard to go to my London haunts, because everything reminded me of drinking. I'd see someone and think, 'I can't spend time with them because I'll want a drink! I have to get out of here.'

Staying sober involves a whole lifestyle change, and the people who don't last are the ones who don't adjust their lifestyle. Normally, when I was going to a social event, I'd think, 'Great, I'll have a few glasses of wine with the girls before we go out.'

But all of that had to end – and although I'm glad it has, because I could never stop at a few glasses of wine, it took time to make the adjustment.

You have to change everything around you – and then you realise who your true friends are. My worry was: 'Oh, my friends will hate that I've stopped.'

Actually, they don't really care. Once you've left, do you think the party will be any less fun for them? Will it buggery!

After about an hour they'll say, 'Did Denise go? Oh, really boring . . . anyway . . .'

No one cares. Everyone is living their own life. Anybody who really cares about you will support you: friends like Carol McGiffin, for instance. Everyone thought, 'Oh, McGiffin will hate the fact that Den's sober! She's lost her drinking buddy.'

But actually Carol was really happy for me, because she saw that I had a problem. Drinking doesn't make Carol depressed, or cause her to crash, or create shame. Whereas it did with me – and that's the difference. That's why Carol was protective when people tried to offer me a drink after I'd stopped, even if she was drinking herself. She wants me to be happy. She's my real friend.

Carol quite openly says, 'Denise doesn't drink any more and I don't drink any less.'

You've got to love that!

People who don't care about you very much will tell you you're boring – and they're the friends where you might have to think, 'Do you know, I don't really need them in my life any more! I'm going to do a bit of a cull.'

It's a great opportunity to trim the fat – and you find you don't have to work very hard at it, because the lukewarm friends don't really want to be around you any more. They were only on your coat-tails because you were the party ringleader.

You have people saying, 'You've given up drinking? Oh God, you're so boring.'

These are the people who don't understand that you had a drink problem. Often, when you're talking to them, you get to a point when you think, 'Oh my God, no, *you're* boring! If only you knew how boring you are.'

Once or twice I've wanted to say so, especially if they've brought it up the next time I've seen them. 'Oh my God, Mrs Boring, you went home really early!' they'll say.

'If we're talking boring, please tell me the story about the missing dog again,' I want to say. 'Fourteen times just wasn't enough.'

But usually I just smile my way through it.

I wish that I could carry around with me a one-way mirror that I could sit behind and watch the carnage that is wrought when there's too much alcohol and people begin to change. You've got your friends who get slurry and repetitive when they drink; the friends who get mean; and the friends who get argumentative. It's really interesting to see the ones who get ultra-flirty, too. But it's not a world that I miss. When you are with the right people, then being sober at a party can be fantastic fun.

The people around me now don't think I'm boring, because I'm not boring. The only people who think you're entertaining when you're drinking are people who are as drunk as you. Sober people don't think you're entertaining, because you're not. You're boring!

I have a close friend who is a binge-drinker like I was. These days she loves being out with me because she stays sober. I don't make her – she just uses the time with me to be sober. She wakes up the next day and thinks, 'Wow, I just love this feeling of waking up clear-headed in the morning!' She's amazed at how much she manages to get done by eleven o'clock.

Not drinking doesn't mean I don't dance, but I don't dance on tables any more. You have to adapt. I'm not going to say it's always a barrel of laughs to be sober in the corner of a packed room where everyone is drinking, but it can be great to go along to a party for two or three hours and then leave, having had a nice time, just at the point when people are beginning to get pissed and perhaps a bit boring or repetitive.

People say, 'You're sober, how brilliant! How many years? You must have had a drink at your wedding to Lincoln, though?'

'Noooo! What part of "I'm sober" do you not understand?' I think. 'If I was the person who could have a couple of drinks at my wedding, I wouldn't be an alcoholic. I wouldn't be sober!'

It drives me mad, but I just smile and say, 'No, I didn't have a drink at my wedding.'

'Yeah, but you'll have a drink at Christmas, won't you?' they say, shuddering at the thought of being sober at a family gathering.

No, I won't, because I don't drink! I won't drink at my niece's wedding or my aunt and uncle's golden wedding anniversary, but I will enjoy myself.

My relationships within the family have improved no end since I got sober. My sister worried about my drinking more than anyone and would certainly be the most vocal about it. Her disapproval of me was evident, which would put up a barrier between us. Now, when I see my sister, we have none of that going on. We still have our moments, but they are not compounded by alcohol.

Most of the time I feel sympathy and compassion for myself when I think back to the days when I was drinking too much, but there are moments when I go cold and feel a sense of disgust. Shame can be a motivator to never go there again – to never be that person again. It is something that only you can overcome – nobody else can do it for you – and I am learning to deal with it. I'm trying to put the past behind me.

Guilt is something we all experience, especially as women and mothers. Should I be working? Should I have sent him to school when he's not well? I should have been there for that sports day and I wasn't because I was working. Guilt, guilt, guilt – everyone has it. When it comes to my children, I have guilt to this day, especially regarding the way they saw me being presented in the media.

Matthew says, 'Mum, the fact is, you gave up drinking and you've given me and Louis wings to fly. If you weren't in the place you are now, I wouldn't be able to travel internationally because I would be worried about you.'

Along with guilt, I have a lot of shame, and it's something that only I can work on. My main regret is that I want to go back and be the person I am now when Matthew was young – and I can't. I just have to come to terms with things and value the fact that I have moved on. It's something that I'm dealing with now: I am having therapy to try to sort out my issues with regret about some of the decisions I made when the children were small. It's about looking after my general mental health, not necessarily my clinical depression.

Matthew has said that he doesn't really remember me being poorly when he was a kid. I think Tim and I protected him from it as much as possible. If you say to a child, 'Mummy's poorly,' she's just poorly. It was never really spelt out to him, but as he got a little bit older I used to say to him, 'I've got my thing,' and he would completely understand.

When I first heard his song, 'She Lays Down' – his version of my illness based on some of the things I told him – I realised that as much as he understands the pain I went through from my perspective, he understands it from his own experiences as well.

I wish I had dealt with my pain differently during Matthew's childhood. I wish I could have the time back, because it definitely impacted on him. He's a wonderful person and he has a global voice that he uses to do such incredible good. He's a champion of so many causes, including women's rights, Amnesty International, the LGBTQ community and other oppressed minorities. Hopefully, he got some of that from me – and obviously from his dad, of course – but he also has anxieties and memories that are based on the dysfunctional days of childhood when I wasn't as mentally present as I should have been.

I cringe when I think of some of the people I invited back to our home. When I see these people out in Alderley Edge today, I think, 'Wow, twenty years later you're still hanging around the same bars, talking the same rubbish,' which shows what kind of people they are.

Still, I had them back to my home and so my kids had to deal with them.

'Mum, if you weren't a bit rock 'n' roll, we wouldn't be the band that we are today,' Matthew says, and there is undoubtedly some truth in that.

But if you have a parent who is self-medicating, there will always be things that you would prefer not to have heard or seen – and I have to take responsibility for that. It was less the case for Louis, who was brought up in a sober household from the age of eleven, but he didn't escape unscathed, either.

Would I do things differently if I could go back? Without a shadow of a doubt, although I would never want to go back to those awful times. But my children were always loved and they look back on their childhoods as being happy, even if there were some bumpy times and I made some mistakes in my parenting. That's not trying to justify the mistakes I made, because I made them and I've had to acknowledge them and do a lot of work on myself. Although I can't redo Matty's childhood, I feel grateful that Tim and I raised two great kids, who love me regardless.

V

My grandpa, my dad's dad, owned a sweetie firm in Whitley Bay called John W. Welch. Grandpa's company made the toffees, boiled sweets and humbugs you found in those big glass jars in sweet shops of old. When I came along a little bit earlier than my parents planned, Grandpa made my dad leave university and become a salesman for the family firm. It was a lifelong regret for Dad, but brilliant for me because it meant I was on the 'A' list of every children's party in the area, as I would always turn up with a big jar of toffees! My friends used to enter my house as if it was Aladdin's cave. They gazed in wonder at the chocolates and sweets that my dad was selling, and called me Truly Scrumptious, after the character in *Chitty Chitty Bang Bang*. But, funnily enough, I didn't have a sweet tooth as a child. In fact, I didn't have a sweet tooth until I gave up drinking eight years ago.

Lincoln and I thought we'd solved our problems when we gave up drinking. Little did we realise that when you have an addictive personality, you automatically reach for something else to replace what you've given up. In our case it was food.

Most people who stop drinking, even just for a dry January, will seek a substitute. It's a combination of things: you feel deprived and want to give yourself a treat; you feel virtuous and think you deserve a treat; and if you've been using alcohol as an emotional crutch – as I did a lot of the time – you need something else to fill the hole. Also, there is a lot of sugar content in alcohol, so your body goes into massive craving mode for sugar.

While I was drinking and smoking, the sweet trolley didn't feature in my life. As soon as dinner was over it was, 'More red wine, thank you, and a cigarette, please.'

I really looked forward to my appetite suppressants after a meal.

When the smoking ban came in, I was outside with all the smokers by the time the sweet trolley came round, with my glass of wine and my fag. Pooh-pooh to the honeycomb cheesecake! It didn't tempt me at all, whereas nowadays I could eat the whole thing.

When people used to ask me, 'What would be your last meal?' or, 'What's your favourite meal?', mine was always a starter and a main course. Dessert never featured. Now, though, if someone asked me that question, I'd start with the dessert! That's how much my tastes have changed.

After we gave up drinking, Lincoln and I would end a meal by saying, 'Let's have something sweet.'

I hadn't given up smoking, and yet was craving sugar like crazy. I couldn't wait for the main course to be over to get to the pudding, and nor could Lincoln.

I could see a couple of pounds going on, but my attitude was, 'Well, I deserve it. I'm not going to worry about a few pounds. Bloody hell, I've given up drinking!'

I had never really bothered very much about weight since a brief frenzy of dieting in my teens, after which I stayed quite slim because of all the bad things in my life. First, I smoked. Then depression kept me slim, because I don't eat during a bad episode. Then came alcohol, which works as a replacement for food, and of course, my past cocaine use, the most famous appetite suppressor of them all.

People would say, 'Your figure looks amazing!' and 'You're so slim!'

I didn't like to say, 'It's because I'm not really eating properly.'

I put on weight quite fast and it wasn't long before I noticed an extra chin when I saw myself on the TV monitors at *Loose Women*. At first, I thought, 'I'm going to have to watch this. I'm looking a bit podgy.'

But my friends were saying, 'No, you're not Densy! Bloody hell, if you can't have a pudding… look at you giving up drinking! You're amazing.'

I did feel incredibly proud of myself, although I wasn't happy about the weight. When I was offered a play, *Smack Family Robinson*, directed by Richard Wilson of *One Foot in the Grave* fame, I said to him, 'I must go on a diet.'

'Darling, you're not dieting on my watch,' he said. 'One of the lines in the play is, "I've got an arse the size of Norfolk," so you'd better not lose any weight.'

'Brilliant,' I thought. 'The director wants me to keep on eating – hurrah!'

It was another excuse to tuck into pudding.

One day while I was doing the play, I was walking over Kingston Bridge, in Surrey, when I lost my balance and fell to my knees. It was mortifying and I was flushed with embarrassment as people ran up to me, asking, 'Are you all right?'

'Yes, oh my goodness, I just tripped. I'm fine!' I said.

One of my knees was very swollen and sore as a result of the fall, and I went to see a specialist doctor in Kingston. He told me that I had severe osteoarthritis in my knees, and particularly in one knee. Was it my left knee? I can't remember, because it's completely okay now.

The doctor asked me about my weight, and I said, 'Well, I . . .'

I was very much in denial about how much I had put on. 'I have gained a little bit of weight since I gave up alcohol,' I said, eventually.

'It's marvellous that you've given up alcohol,' he said, beaming. 'How much weight have you gained?'

I got on the scales. The moment had come when I had to face the fact that I was over two stone heavier than before. On a small frame like mine, at five foot four, it's a lot. I wasn't ten stone overweight, so it wasn't a horrendous obesity problem, but I was potentially on the way to obesity, because I was finding it hard to pull back.

The shock of weighing myself gave me pause for thought and I realised that I was eating in the way that I used to drink – not when I was depressed, necessarily, but when I was low and pissed off and fed up. Instead of having a glass of wine, I was eating, and not only was I eating massive amounts of carbs and chocolate, I was also secret eating.

I didn't sneak around eating secretly because Lincoln and Louis watched what I was eating. They didn't say, 'Don't you have any chocolate before bed!'

It was shame that made me secretive. I felt bad that I couldn't control my appetite. I would have a pudding or dessert with Louis and Lincoln, and then I'd sneak out and have another piece of cheesecake later. If they came into the kitchen while I was munching, I'd be like the cartoon character with chocolate around my mouth, trying to look innocent.

'What have you been doing?'

'Nothing!'

It's comical when I tell the story, but in fact it was desperately unhealthy. I was getting chocolate bars and quickly eating them on my own. I wasn't sitting down, being present and enjoying the chocolate as I ate it, which is how I would eat it now: I was stuffing it in guiltily and compulsively. I was yet to learn that there's nothing wrong with having a chocolate bar or a big pasta treat or a generous portion of fish and chips when you make an informed decision to eat it.

Within a year of giving up drinking, I had put on over two stone. Lincoln had proposed to me and we had set the date for our wedding for 13 July 2013, so I felt I had to lose weight, fast. It was April and I was getting married in July.

By now, I was making self-deprecating jokes about my weight so that nobody could get in first and say something hurtful. It was the same approach that I'd had when I played the part of 'Drunk Spice' on *Loose Women* and tried to pre-empt the newspapers printing a photo of me coming out of a nightclub. Instead of being embarrassed by what the papers printed, I'd be on *Loose Women* saying, 'Yes, I was out until 4 in the morning, so what? Just because I'm in my late forties doesn't mean you can't have a bloody good time, does it, audience? Wahay!'

I did the same with my weight gain and tried to get in there first before the papers said, 'Look at Denise!'

So, if a guest came on the show and they were really slim, I'd say, 'Don't sit her next to me, it will show up how big I am, haha!'

At the same time, I had to be careful not to offend people watching the show who were morbidly obese, and who would think that my weight gain was minimal.

'Can we do a topic about putting on weight and how we all deal with it, so that I can talk about it in a constructive way?' I asked the team at *Loose Women*. 'Can I say that I feel as if my eating has taken the place of drinking in my life?'

Loose Women can be a marvellous vehicle for tackling this kind of topic. It's why the programme is so important, because we're the only show on television where we, the presenters, reveal our vulnerable sides. Normally, presenters don't talk about their politics, their feelings about relationships or their marriages. It's quite nerve-racking at times, but it can be a very positive thing.

Talking openly on television about my desire to lose weight

led several diet companies to get in touch. They saw it as an opportunity to push their product, because they're all businesspeople, of course.

Lincoln was helping me with a few of my projects and said, 'Let's sit down and see which is the best diet for you.'

Of course, I knew how to diet; I knew that if I put fewer calories in my mouth, I would lose weight. However, it's not as simple as that; the important thing is to maintain your weight, moving forward. The reason that we chose LighterLife was that the focus was as much on changing your relationship with food using Cognitive Behavioural Therapy (CBT) as it was on losing weight.

It had already dawned on me that if I didn't change my approach to eating, I would spend a lifetime battling my weight, yo-yo dieting, stressing about it, emotional eating and using food as a crutch, in the same way I had done with alcohol. I felt that CBT was offering me a lifeline and I grabbed it. That's why I decided to form an allegiance with LighterLife and become their ambassador.

It took willpower, but I lost two stone in two months, which is exactly what it said on the tin. Not only did I feel amazing, from an aesthetic point of view, because I was slim again, but I also felt an improvement in my breathing and my snoring. And when I saw a joint specialist in Cheshire, I was told that my osteoarthritis had improved by 90%! That was a result of losing two stone, so you can imagine the burden on the joints of people who are five or ten stone overweight.

I now work with a lot of people with weight issues and it breaks my heart when I see the cycle they're trapped in, because it's the same cycle I was in with drink and drugs. They feel so down and so low in self-esteem that they hate themselves. So, what do they do? They eat.

There is a myth that you should lose weight slowly. People

say, 'She has lost weight far too quickly,' or, 'I can't believe he has lost so much, far too quickly.'

When I first put on weight, the weekly women's magazines said, 'Densy is celebrating her curves,' and 'Denise shows off her fuller figure.'

Then, when I lost it, the headline was, 'You've gone too far!'

The idea that slow weight loss was better came from a paper that was published in the Sixties and has since been disproved, and yet we're still saying it, even though it makes no sense at all. In my experience, people tell you not to lose weight too quickly for the same reason your piss-head friends don't want you to stop drinking, because your sobriety is highlighting their drink problem. Those are the people you trim from your life, ideally.

Nobody wants to lose a pound a month. Rapid weight loss works – it can reverse Type 2 diabetes in people! It doesn't just arrest the disease, it gets rid of it. And as you lose the weight, CBT can help teach you how to change your relationship with food.

CBT sounds complex, but it gives you simple tools to combat your behaviour. Take Jessie, for instance. Jessie is overweight, and she is trying to lose the excess. She uses food as a crutch when she's happy and also when she's low, sad, down in the dumps and disappointed about life. One day, Jessie comes home after a really horrible day at work. She thinks, 'I am going to order a big, fuck-off, takeaway pizza because that is the only thing I know will comfort me.'

The CBT approach to her situation would be as follows: 'Jessie, when you feel this way, as low as you're feeling, just try and take one minute, just 60 seconds, to think it through. You'll order the pizza and it will come within half an hour. When it comes, you will probably shovel it in your mouth and it will all be gone within ten minutes. So, within the next hour, you will have shoved it in your mouth and you'll be left with the grease dripping down your chin.

'How are you going to feel when that has happened, Jessie? Are you going to feel amazing? Will you feel that your mood has lifted? Is your bullying boss going to stop bullying you?

'No, Jessie, you're going to feel worse. You're going to feel disgusted at yourself. You're going to ask yourself, "Why did I do that? Because now, I've got indigestion, my breathing is impaired again and I feel like shit, because I don't have the willpower to say no to that pizza. I'm just a waste of space."'

CBT gives you an alternative. It teaches you to think, 'Okay, I'm hungry, and I'm going to eat, and I'm going to go to the fridge and I'm going to make myself something really tasty and nutritious, and I'm going to eat it. It may not be as gorgeous, going in, as that pizza, but when I've finished it and my tummy is full, I'm going to think, "Bloody good for you, Jessie!" I'm going to start feeling that I'm more in control of my life, because I made a healthy decision.'

I see a lot of people who encourage their partners to drink, and there are food enablers, too. Take John, for instance: I'll say, 'John, hang on a minute, she's trying to lose weight, she doesn't want the pudding.'

'Oh, she loves a bit of banoffee pie,' John says.

'Yes, but she's trying to lose weight, John. Support her in this journey. Don't put the banoffee pie down in front of her.'

John doesn't like how Susie is changing, because John is losing control and Susie is gaining control; she is looking amazing and John is worried and jealous. It doesn't mean that John is a bad person, but John wants her to have the banoffee pie and keep things as they were.

I see this scenario quite often. A perfect example was Paula, a woman in my weight loss group. Paula had been 20 stone, and ten stone was her target. She reached her target during my time in the group and I was there when we celebrated her ten stone weight. She looked amazing. Oh my God, the joy on her face was unbelievable.

I kept in touch with Paula, and we all met up for a coffee a few months later. Paula had put on some weight, after being bullied by her family. She had lost ten stone and become, in theory, a different person, physically and mentally. Suddenly, her mother-in-law was worried that Paula would cheat on her husband, because that's what Paula's sister-in-law had done with her husband's brother.

'You're doing the same thing, I can tell,' the mother-in-law kept saying. 'Why are you losing weight? He likes you as you are. We've never said anything to you about your weight. It's because you're having an affair, isn't it? And if you're not now, you will do. Who do you think you are?'

This underlying pattern of control and enabling is very common. Unhappiness makes people eat because their family don't want them to change their lives and upset the status quo. It's very hard for people, especially if they are fat shamed. Often people are fat because they're desperately unhappy.

Of course, not everybody has to be thin and a size ten. I'm a size 12 and sometimes a 14 top because of my boobs. I'm not a skinny Lizzy; I've got bumps and curves. But I know how to maintain my weight for my health, because I have been given the tools to do so, and I'm forever grateful for that, because they are tools for life.

I am still that person that wants to comfort eat when I'm down, of course I am. Do I still comfort eat, sometimes?

Of course I do, but I also know how to stop doing it.

We are all frail; we can't resist temptation all the time. I've fallen off the wagon a couple of times, but it's okay, because I have the tools to get back on it again.

PART 5

A New Life

I

Two years ago, I was sitting on the beach in Grenada, eating apple pie in the sunshine, with palm trees swaying above me and waves lapping at my feet, when the colour began to bleed away from my surroundings and my hands started to tingle.

'You're not well, are you?' Lincoln said.

'No,' I said.

Within seconds, the unwelcome visitor had arrived.

It was early January, and in the weeks and days leading up to this moment, I had been driving Lincoln mad with my tidy obsession. Ours is not a massive house, and Lincoln keeps most of his things at his studio – Lincoln, by the way, is now a contemporary artist, but inevitably stuff accumulates. I don't worry too much about it when I'm well, but when I'm poorly all I want is clean surfaces and an absence of clutter. So, instead of making Lincoln and Louis laugh by saying, 'Anybody want any of these 19,000 pairs of unworn trainers that are spilling out of the office?' I'll snipe, 'Lincoln, I've asked you a million times to clear up the shoes . . .'

I think he knows it's a sign that I'm getting poorly and it makes him a bit prickly. 'Darling, I can either sell a painting or I can do the shoes,' he says.

Since I'm not normally a nag, it's a different 'me' that says, 'Darling, these brochures . . .'

'Yes, they're going to the studio,' he says curtly.

'Okay, it's just that you said that, you know, last week . . .'

When I'm on holiday, I find solace in living clutter-free. I love having a capsule wardrobe that I mix and match every day. 'I could live with just these clothes, all the time!' I think.

I'll wear the same pair of shoes every day, so there's none of the bother of 'Where are my boots?' that I have back at home.

'Isn't it lovely living with only a capsule wardrobe?' I kept saying to Lincoln in Grenada. 'I much prefer it.'

'Well, why not chuck some clothes out when you get home?' he suggested. 'You've got twenty-seven wardrobes full of stuff.'

'I'll get a skip when we get back,' I said.

'For your clothes?' Lincoln asked.

'No, I've decided I'm going to clear all the boxes and stuff out of the little room under the stairs, because I can't stand the thought of all that mess being there.

'Do you remember the guy we bought the house from? He kept the room under the stairs so tidy, with all his DVDs lined up on the shelves. So I was thinking, if I get a skip . . .'

Under the palm trees, I was transported by visions of other people's tidy houses and clean surfaces.

'Where's your clutter?' I always ask when I go to someone's house. 'Where is it?'

'In the drawers and cupboards,' they say.

But if you open one of their drawers, it's as neat as the rest of the house. 'Where are your overstuffed cupboards that don't close?' I screech. 'Where's the key drawer that doesn't have any keys in it?'

'Yes, a skip is definitely the answer . . .' I mused aloud to Lincoln.

'We're on holiday in the Caribbean! Let it go with the skip,' he begged.

The problem is, I'm a tidy person trapped in the body of somebody who's quite untidy. I hate domesticity, clearing, tidying and lifting; there's always something else more interesting to do. So although I want to be the person who has no clutter, when I have a day free, I can't face doing it. It's so boring, so tedious. I'd rather sneak back into my bedroom with my cuppa and watch rubbish TV on my phone!

'I'm not going down there now,' I think. 'I'll do it another day.'

I'll never know whether the unwelcome visitor was coming anyway while we were on holiday, or whether stress had lowered my defences over Christmas, leaving the door open for him to come in. It had not been a festive season for me: I'd had a horrible situation with a pantomime production company in Newcastle; they had fired me from my role in *Jack and the Beanstalk* amidst a dispute about safety concerns, staff wage issues, technical problems and a disastrous level of preparation for opening night. It was incredibly traumatic, because the papers initially reported that I'd walked away, like some kind of diva. People thought I had let down thousands of people in my home town by walking out of a pantomime, which was untrue and upsetting. I've never walked away from anything.

After a horrendous time involving lawyers, I was completely exonerated. The pantomime closed early owing thousands of pounds. The upside of this debacle was that I got to go to Grenada in early January, where, apart from my obsession with neatness, we were having a blissful time. Maybe there were other signs that the visitor was on his way, though. The night before he came, I didn't feel very well and didn't want to go to dinner. It made me feel guilty, because it meant Lincoln had to go along on his own.

Sometimes a tummy ache can be a warning that the visitor is close. But I'm never sure. Is it psychosomatic? Is it an actual tummy ache? Or a sign of not wanting to do something?

'Don't worry, I'll go on my own,' Lincoln said.

'But . . .'

'It's not the end of the world. I'm hungry, darling. Do you want anything to eat?'

'No, thanks.'

I wasn't hungry. It was another sign, but I didn't connect it to becoming poorly.

We were staying in quite a small, exclusive resort, and after breakfast the next morning, we went over to the beach bar area to sunbathe. I had booked a teacher to come every day and show us how to do yoga, and we were about to go off to our yoga class in a beautiful, open-air lodge.

I was trying to be good with my diet, but of course the resort owner came over and said, 'You've got to try our home-made apple pie and cream.'

I was halfway through my apple pie when I felt it starting: black cloud, joy going, tinny taste, tingling hands. 'I don't want to be here, don't want to be with anyone, don't want to talk to anybody or eat anything. I'm poorly,' I thought, putting down my plate.

We were five or six days into a twelve-day trip and I wasn't well enough to go to yoga again. Lincoln still went and I felt really guilty about it, even though he never once said, 'You should be coming with me.'

'What did you say to the teacher?' I asked.

'I just said you weren't very well, and you're not,' Lincoln said.

Later in the day I phoned Matthew. When I'm not well, I need everyone I love to realise how poorly I am, so that they will check up on me, because I think that if they ring me it'll make me feel better. It's not good to rely on people to make me feel okay, but that's what happens.

Matthew was duly sympathetic, but when he hadn't rung me by three o'clock the next day, I sent him a reproachful text. He interpreted the text as if I was doubting his love for me, which I wasn't, and yet when I'm poorly everything gets

mushed up with my guilt about his childhood. It's complicated! We sorted it out, though. Usually he just sends me a
picture of Livia, Tony's mother in *The Sopranos*, when he
thinks I'm putting pressure on him to reply to my calls. (She's
the one who's always saying, 'You don't call, you don't
write . . . what's going on?')

The visitor stayed for three days, and then he left. I was fine
for the last three days of the holiday. It was as if nothing had
happened.

My depression tends to lift during the day. At the end of my
most recent episode, Lincoln and I were at home and I was on
the sofa in my sloth position watching TV when I felt the visitor starting to go. I kept quiet, like a child hoping that if I
stayed still and silent, I would become invisible to my parents
and they would forget it was time for bath and bed.

Was he really leaving?

I said nothing to Lincoln. I didn't want to get his hopes up.

I went into the kitchen to make a cup of coffee. I'm only a
Gold Blend drinker – I'm hardly a frappuccino lover – but
when I'm poorly, my desire for coffee is the first thing that
goes. If it's back, it can often mean that I'm getting better.

I also know I'm poorly when I don't want to watch any of
my favourite American reality shows. To test myself, I'll think
about watching TV with Lincoln and, if it feels like quite a
nice thing to do, I'll know the visitor is on his way out.

Sometimes I ask myself how I feel about the ironing that's
piling up in the utility room. I don't do my ironing, because
we're lucky enough to have Christine to do it, so it shouldn't
really stress me. But when I'm poorly, it suddenly matters.
Meanwhile, if I think, 'I'm not bothered about the ironing,' it
means I'm getting better.

I watch the unwelcome visitor retreat with bated breath. Is
he going to turn around, like an evil villain, and say, 'A-ha, I
fooled you! I'm not really leaving after all'?

I often won't tell anyone he's going until much later in the day, or the next morning – until the door actually slams and he has gone.

Sometimes I cry when he has left. Not boo-hoo crying – just crying with relief. It's like being trapped under a boulder, not knowing how long you're going to be under there, until a rescue squad lifts it off you.

My friends Pam, Ange and Rose came to see me during my most recent episode. (Fortunately, Pam was still speaking to me after I had mistakenly thrown a box of her precious heirlooms out during one of my cleaning blitzes – but that's another story!) Pam, Ange and Rose knew I was poorly and came to show they cared. My friends are very understanding. They say, 'Is there anything we can do?' and stay for just a short time.

I want to withdraw when I'm poorly, but paradoxically, if I don't see anyone, it makes me feel worse. 'I'm now becoming completely reclusive,' I think. So we try to keep some kind of normality going.

Not being poorly themselves, Pam, Ange and Rose were chatting about the usual things. Normally, I love my friends coming round and I'm fascinated by everything they have to say, but when I'm depressed, nothing interests me, so I couldn't engage. 'I want to be interested, but I'm not,' I thought. 'I just want to be on my own.'

Of course, after the visitor had gone, I wanted them to come back and tell me their stories all over again.

There are times when, just like everyone else, I don't answer my phone, especially if I'm in the middle of a *Love After Lockup* double episode, which will always take precedence over everything. If my agent, Bex, rings though, I always pick up. Any actor will understand that when I see Bex's name come up on my phone, my tummy tips over, because it might be 'that' movie! In any case, I've got a great friendship with Bex and we talk about Louis's acting career quite a lot, as she looks after Louis as well.

I drive her mad about Louis, actually. We joke that I mustn't do a Kris Jenner, the Kardashian mother, who coined the phrase 'momager'. Now that Louis is nineteen, it's, 'Butt out, Mother!' unless she can't get hold of him.

I'll say, 'I'm not being Kris Jenner, but . . .'

'I've spoken to him and to *Emmerdale*. It's got nothing to do with you,' Bex replies firmly, emailing me a picture of Kris Jenner.

When I'm poorly, I don't answer the phone to anybody, not even Bex. The sound of my phone ringing makes me jump and the thought of having a discussion appals me.

'I know you're not well because you're not taking my calls,' Bex will say.

She's always on the alert for it. Even if I'm just quiet because I'm doing something else, she'll ring me and say, 'Are you okay?'

Everyone close to me is aware that when I'm ill I withdraw from their life.

For years, the book I always kept by my bed was Spike Milligan's account of his depression, based on his conversations with Dr Anthony Clare. Milligan described the illness as I felt it. At last I had found a book about depression that I could relate to.

Just knowing that Milligan had my illness helped me. He wasn't telling me how to get better. He wasn't better himself. And yet, throughout the book he maintained his sense of humour. He talked about how his illness affected his personal life, but also highlighted the times when he managed to work while feeling poorly, with the Goons among others. I empathised, I sympathised and I laughed along. It was a huge solace to me, and an inspiration to keep working and pushing through.

One of Spike Milligan's main triggers was conflict within his family. If his daughters were arguing with each other, or if his wife was arguing with his daughters, it could set off a massive decline in him and then a deep depression, which could last for as long as eighteen months. I understood this, because I hate conflict in my family. It can unsettle me and make me very anxious, and I have to work hard at talking my way out of it.

If I feel the unwelcome visitor coming because of conflict within the family, I'll say to him, 'Don't come. Let me deal with this. It's only an argument, for God's sake! People have arguments every single day. Why would my family never have an argument? Of course they argue. All families argue.'

This is what is going on in my head as I try to make him go away again, and sometimes it will work. I will sense him walking up the path, but he never gets to the door.

If he comes in and shuts the door behind him, he's there until he decides to leave, and there's nothing I can do. Talking therapy won't make a difference. Hot baths don't help and neither does mindfulness. When it's in my system – when whatever happens has changed my body chemistry and caused the depression – it has to undo itself, physically, before I start feeling better.

It's very hard because if anything tests your sobriety, it's depression. You want something to change your mood, but I have nothing, because I don't drink or do drugs.

In America, people who know I have depression say to me, 'Why don't you try edibles?' (They mean edible marijuana, which is legal in some states in America.)

'Because I don't do drugs!' I say.

I can't have anything that changes how I feel, and I don't want to. I want to be able to deal with life myself. Also, if I did try edibles and they worked, I would inevitably become reliant on them and have another battle on my hands. Since I have no off-button, the old hash brownies would be coming out at breakfast! I could never risk it.

I don't want to be the drink police, or any other kind of police. My sobriety doesn't mean I'm against people having a good time. I'm just saying to those people who have a propensity to depression and anxiety, if you take alcohol out of your life, it is a better life. You still have the illness, but you enjoy the times in between episodes much more, and you're not compounding it when you're in it.

II

I have completely accepted that my depression is an illness I have for life and that it will always return. So why I keep agreeing to do live theatre is anybody's guess! I think I must have this desire to keep reminding people that I'm an award-winning actress, even though I'm sometimes putting myself through hell to do it. There are a lot of people in this industry who suffer from anxiety and depression, and many of them have avoided theatre for years because it's so terrifying. It's bad enough getting ill when you are filming, but it's nightmarish to get it when you're onstage.

Before I did *Little Voice* at the Manchester Royal Exchange in 2004, there had been a period of several years when I wouldn't do theatre, because I was just too frightened. But there's something in me that won't allow the unwelcome visitor to ruin my life any more than he has. While I was at drama school, I had dreamt of working with the Royal Exchange Theatre Company, and with *Little Voice* I was determined to face my fear of having an episode onstage. Thankfully, it was a monster success. That's what the papers said: '*Little Voice* is a monster success.' It was sold out for every single performance and lots of industry people came to see it.

The run finished on a Saturday night. Just before we went on for the Saturday matinee, the penultimate performance, someone said, 'Chris Eccleston's in,' and he's an actor I admired hugely, and still do.

Quite early on in the matinee, as the words of the play were coming out of my mouth, I thought, 'Wouldn't it be awful if I got my thing before I finished the run?'

Instantly, it started – and I dried.

It's horrible thinking about it, because I can still feel that paralysing fear. When you dry onstage, it is probably only ten seconds at the most before you either remember the line or another actor gets you out of it, but it feels like a year. Panic filled my body, and although the line eventually came back to me, I gave the rest of my performance in a state of anxiety.

Non-actors often think the big challenge of doing theatre is remembering your lines, but when you've been doing a play for a while, and if you're enjoying the performance, remembering your lines isn't really an issue. In a fantastic play like *Little Voice*, the only reason you forget your lines is if you lose concentration, which might happen if your mind strays and you don't listen and follow the text, so don't know when to come in – or it might happen if something is happening to you, as it was to me. I was panicking and my ears were ringing; I was in a state of internal chaos and in fear of my illness coming. Then it came with a whoosh, and it was terrifying having to mask it with 700 faces staring at me.

Actors have three versions of the same nightmare: being onstage and not knowing your lines; not knowing the play; or being naked onstage.

Every actor has them. First, you hear the stage manager say, 'It's *Beginners*.'

'But I don't know the play. I don't know the words!' you cry.

'How is that possible? We've all been rehearsing for three weeks!'

'But I don't know it. What have we been rehearsing?'

Suddenly, you're onstage, without a clue about anything.

With my illness, the real-life actor's nightmare would happen to me, but worse. Yet I've never considered giving up acting. I know people who have left this profession because they suffer from depression, but there was always a part of me that would not let the visitor ruin my career.

I was prepared to fight him every time. I'd think, 'If you're coming onstage with me, fucking come, but you'll see that I won't run off the stage.'

And I never did, although I've come pretty damn close to it a couple of times.

When Chris Eccleston came backstage after the performance, he was full of compliments. He hadn't noticed anything at all. Afterwards, I went into my dressing room and screamed, 'You were there all the time, but I still did it, and Chris Eccleston said I was good, despite you, you bastard! So, come on, I dare you. Come at me again.' It sounds mad, but that's what I did.

Each time I am presented with a massive challenge during an episode and I push through it, it helps me get through the next time. I've had to push through on many occasions when I was acting – and occasionally in social situations, too. I had a very tough time in 2015 when I did *The Ancient Secret of Youth and the Five Tibetans*, a new Jim Cartwright play at the Octagon Theatre in Bolton. The unwelcome visitor was with me every day through rehearsals – every day, through a three-week rehearsal period – and I was playing the lead. It was hardcore.

By then I had stepped back from *Loose Women*. I needed a break from the show where I was sharing so much of my life; it was time to re-evaluate everything, now that I had given up drinking. I also wanted to focus on my acting career, so I was hugely flattered to be asked to be in the play, which I loved the moment I read it. It helped that the theatre was near my home, a 45-minute drive, but mainly I was thrilled to be working with a director I'd always wanted to work with, in a theatre I'd always wanted to work at, with a company of players I admired.

Everything about it was enjoyable. I wasn't stressed or anxious at all.

During the very early stages of rehearsal, my depression came on endogenously, like it does, for no reason that I'm aware of. I woke up one morning and it was there. It was grey depression, as opposed to black depression, and I can work through grey depression – but it took every bit of fun out of the rehearsal period.

Unfortunately, when it wouldn't lift, I couldn't take myself to bed and remove myself from pressure, be looked after and soothe myself. There was only a very small section of the play when I wasn't onstage. That's a real pressure when you're in theatre and have no understudy. I couldn't have a day off. And so the visitor stayed.

It's very hard when you're playing the lead in something, but in the end, I did take a day off. My excuse was that I was physically poorly. The company manager rang me. 'You will be back tomorrow though, Den, won't you? Because there's so little that we can do without you.'

I didn't tell anyone that I was depressed. I felt a duty of care to all the cast and thought that if my cast-mates started worrying that I was mentally ill, they would lose their trust in me. Actors are dependent on each other onstage, and for your own safety as an actor, you need to be able to trust the people around you.

My depression was crippling on the first night. I don't know to this day how I went on, or how I didn't just run away. On nights like these, I think, 'Dear God, I'd like everyone in the world to feel what I'm going through now for fifteen seconds.'

Then everyone in the world would know that depression is one of the worst conditions you can have.

It was debilitating for the whole first half. Thankfully I felt it starting to lift in the second act, probably because the show was going really well. 'I'm getting through it. I'm getting through it. I'm getting through it,' I thought.

Gradually, over the next few days, it got better, and this is where you've got to wonder about the psychology of it. My fear of doing the play with the visitor hovering in the wings was keeping the depression in my system. And I couldn't do anything to try to feel better: I couldn't be kind to myself and empty my diary, which would always be my advice to other people in this situation. Sometimes it's just not possible.

Since no one in the medical profession completely understands my illness, I shouldn't beat myself up for not completely understanding it either, but I do. I just wish I knew what was going on and why, because although my illness has a life of its own, inasmuch as the majority of the time I'm not in control of when it descends, what is happening in my life also seems to play a massive part in it.

When I'm trying to find a reason for why I have depression, I think of the statistics that say very creative people tend to suffer from it more than others. So maybe there's a sensitivity gene in creative people? Who knows? Then again, my illness has hormonal origins and began with having a baby; sensitivity didn't have anything to do with it. Did that first episode open my system up to lifelong depression? Did I already have a sensitivity? It's a weird one. If they knew the answers, medical scientists would be able to cure this illness, but they can't. Thank God they can make it easier with medication.

When I was offered the role of Celia in *Calendar Girls: The Musical*, in 2018, it took me weeks to decide whether or not to do it. My indecision stemmed from the knowledge that I would be attached to the project for ten months and therefore was bound to get poorly at some point, because it is very rare that I go ten months without an episode.

It helped that I had a great understudy, Vanessa Grace Lee, who was there for me professionally and personally. But it was a big role and I was frightened about being ill onstage. 'At what point in the production will I get poorly?' I kept wondering.

There were other considerations. Did I want to be away from home for so long? Did I want to be away from my family, even though they were all doing their own thing anyway? Was I going to miss a TV role that I would regret?

In the end, it was too good an opportunity to miss. It's a great piece of theatre and audiences everywhere loved it; I can't remember a single performance that didn't get a standing ovation. Nevertheless, with every week that went by, whether it was a good week, a bad week, or a not-so-great audience, whether I was having problems with a couple of cast members, or any of the normal things that happen on tour, I kept thinking, 'I wonder if I'll get to the end of this without my thing.'

Whatever I'm doing, it's always in the back of my mind. 'Will I get to the end of this without the visitor coming?'

It was pretty awful when it happened, because of course he did come, out of the blue, after I'd had a sickness bug and a nasty head cold. It was incredibly frightening, one of the most frightening times I've had onstage since *And A Nightingale Sang*, because it happened during the show. If the visitor comes on with me at the beginning of the show, I can usually cope. It's so much worse if he suddenly appears when I'm already onstage.

The show had a big cast and they had all been down with colds and flu, which is inevitable when you have that many people working, touring and living together. But if everybody took time off when they had cold and flu symptoms, there'd be nobody onstage, so after a couple of days off you tend to go back sooner than you should, because you feel guilty. Saying that, one night we had six understudies on and still got a standing ovation! That put paid to any arrogance we had about our individual importance.

I missed a couple of shows in Dublin but had rallied by the time we got to Dartford, although I couldn't shake my head cold and couldn't hear properly. I felt particularly grotty in the second week at Dartford, but I didn't miss a show. By then, we had been touring for six months.

At an evening performance in Dartford, I walked onstage feeling a weird detachment from everything. It was reminiscent of the old feeling of being in a bubble with everything going on around me. 'You're all right. You're all right, you're all right,' I told myself. 'It's just because you've got this head cold. It's not your thing. He's not coming.'

There was a bit where I sang two lines, and as the line was coming up, I started thinking, 'I don't know it!'

The first line came out okay, but I blanked on the second line and just sang, 'La, la, la, la, la, la, la!'

It made the other people on stage corpse. I would have laughed too if it had been somebody else, but I was gripped with anxiety and fear. It was really early on in the show and the production was an ensemble piece where we batted lines between us with quick-fire precision. How was I going to keep going?

I got through the first half. In my dressing room during the interval, I did a piece into my phone, saying, 'I've got my thing. He's here. I'm video recording this. I'm in Dartford and I've just done the first half of the show. I feel terrible and now I've got to get through the second half, with my thing.'

I don't know if I posted it or not, but I intended to, because I wanted to show my depression happening in real time. It was the first time it had occurred to me to do it.

I went back onstage, dreading the scene leading up to my song, because Celia leads that scene. While the words were coming out of my mouth, I grew convinced that I couldn't remember my song lyrics. I was terrified. 'There's only an hour until the end,' I kept telling myself. 'You've got an hour. You've got an hour. You've got an hour.'

My character was a really sassy woman and my song was about empowering older women to do what they want. The audience always loved it when she admitted that she'd had a little work done to her boobs. The message was, 'Do what you want to do, be who you want to be. If you want to get your tits done, get your tits done.'

It was a comic song and as it ended I stood on a chair and sang a loud, long, triumphant note, while the audience whooped and cheered. It was bizarre to hear their laughter and appreciation. 'You have got no idea what I am feeling inside,' I thought.

What made it worse was that I had a friend in to see the show that day, a fellow sufferer, who'd had a breakdown after being sacked from a TV show in the horrible, unceremonious way that people lose their jobs these days. 'Ian's here,' I kept thinking. 'He's been so looking forward to coming to see this show and now it's all going wrong.'

The play went on and we got to the part where we were about to do the famous calendar photoshoot. I looked over at Karen Dunbar, one of my friends among the cast, and caught her eye. 'Are you okay?' she mouthed.

I shook my head.

Karen mimed taking a breath.

'Keep breathing, keep breathing, keep breathing,' I told myself.

For the rest of the show, I used Karen as my guide. She knew what I was going through, having experienced depression and anxiety herself, and looking to her for reassurance got me through the last twenty minutes. It was as if there was Karen, and next to her was the unwelcome visitor; they were both onstage, the devil and my guardian angel, and I was ignoring the devil to look at Karen.

Every line I said, every laugh I got, I looked at her and she winked at me. In my mind, her wink was saying, 'You see? The fucker's with you, but you're still doing it.'

I got to the end of the show and ran offstage. Karen ran off after me, followed by Sara Crowe and AJ Casey, two other friends in the cast. I passed Phil Corbitt, who played John, in the corridor. 'Are you all right?' he asked.

'No!'

I ran into my dressing room and collapsed. I was shaking, crying, panicking and in a terrible, terrible state. It was awful.

'Thank you,' I managed to say to Karen, as she and the others tried to comfort me.

She had helped me through one of the worst moments of my life and nobody out in the audience was any the wiser.

III

One of the things that sobriety has restored to me is my self-esteem. It's funny, because having low self-esteem wasn't something I would ever have admitted to, but, boy, did I have it. I was aware of the way people looked at me at industry dos. They weren't being mean or unfair; they were just sober. I know what I was like at industry dos and when I see people in the same situation now, I feel sorry for them.

Sobriety has brought a sense of massive calm to my life, in between my episodes. It has enabled me to have the most wonderful relationship with my husband. Even in the midst of all our madness, as we call our lives before giving up alcohol, Lincoln and I saw something in each other that was special. It was potentially being ruined by our behaviour, but taking the bad things out of our life has given us a wonderful clarity. It has enabled Lincoln to launch a fantastic career in art that, had he continued drinking, would never have even been a twinkle in his eye. He has turned something he was naturally good at into an international career.

Sobriety has helped me to have a much better relationship with my children. Louis was young when I stopped drinking, so he has grown up, in the main, in a sober household. We all often joke that Matthew's band, the 1975, wouldn't exist if they had been forming during my time with Lincoln. We wouldn't have had teenagers walking through the house at three in the morning! Not when we were in bed by eleven, watching true crime and having a crumpet! It just wouldn't have happened. Our house used to be a bit crazy and was always full of people, and that spawned the 1975 and they're doing very well. All the same, if I had a magic wand, I would like to redo a lot of Matt's childhood.

I try to think, 'You shouldn't have regrets,' but I think it's human nature to have regrets. I regret that my mum didn't live long enough to see my sober life. I regret that I wasn't sober during some of Matt's childhood, when my life was a bit out there. That doesn't mean that I was rolling around the floor – I wasn't that type of drinker – but I wasn't as present as I should have been. Now, though, although my children are grown up, they still need their parents for as long as they're lucky enough to have them, and sobriety has enabled me to have a much clearer perspective on my parenting skills.

Although my depression came many, many times when alcohol wasn't involved, it was just that much worse when I had a hangover. Now, whenever I have an episode, I know that there's nothing I could have done differently. I never have to beat myself up, thinking, 'Oh God, I've got my thing. Here he comes. Why did I have that drink last night?'

I'm back on *Loose Women* now, after a six-year break, and loving it. I get on with all the girls and there are so many things I can talk about that can help others. The team at *Loose Women* are very happy to give me the reins when we do a show on mental health issues. *Loose Women* has played an important role in talking about mental health, for women and for men. Yes, a lot of men watch the show! They may not admit it, but they do.

Being in a completely different place means I'm much more in control of who I am on *Loose Women*. I still end up on the *Mail Online* website for things I say, but the difference is that I know what I'm saying and I believe what I'm saying. As I've said, I would really struggle to look back on those old 'Drunk Spice' episodes, because back then I had completely different views on life, relationships, fidelity and all of the things that are hugely important to me now. Or was it just that I was desperately unhappy?

I'm not saying I was always depressed. Unhappy and depressed are two separate things. When you're depressed, you don't have the ability to be unhappy or happy. There is just a void. I was drinking because I was unhappy and it was compounding my depression, so I was in a mess. Was I 'a functioning alcoholic'? It depends how you define 'functioning'. I don't think I was. Was I turning up for work? Yes. Did I still give good performances? Yes. You can only remain relevant at sixty-two if you've had a successful professional career, never been late, always turned up and done good things. But inside I wasn't functioning.

Still, I'm very proud that I've still got the same friends I've had since my childhood and since I was at drama school. I've always been very popular and loved within my friendship group; I was never somebody who became nasty with drink. The only people I used to push out against were close friends and family who tried to address my drinking, but I was never one of those drinkers who turns on people. Maybe if I had been, I would have stopped earlier, but because I was quite fun to be around, even though I was desperately ill inside, I never lost friends because of my drinking. In fact, I gained them. I was always a nice and kind person, so it's not as if my drinking ever alienated people, even though it was really bad for me.

IV

People say to me, 'Oh my God, you're still posing in a bikini at sixty-two!'

Well, I wouldn't have done it in my forties: I didn't have the confidence in myself then and didn't think people would want to look at me. Why is it different now? I'm not setting myself up as a role model, but I'm a real woman's woman.

It's not, 'Hey, look at me, don't I look fab?' I'm saying, 'I will not be dictated to by the press or by horrible trolls on social media as to whether I should be wearing a bikini at sixty-two. If I can do it, you can do it.'

I don't think I look at all bad for a 62-year-old woman. Yes, I've got a tummy: I've had two children. Yes, I'm a size 12, not a size 8. Yes, I've got a bum and I've got cellulite on my thighs, but I don't think I look bad, and that's because I'm now in control of who I am. That is basically my message.

It really does something for me when I see posts from women, saying, 'We love you, Denise. I was feeling really down on myself today, but now I'm going to put my bikini on and walk along the beach.'

If people want to look on me as an inspiration, then I want to give them inspiration. It's all for the women. That's what I love. I'm not doing it for men to say, 'Cor, what a cracker, Nana!'

I'm not doing it for that. My bikini posts are quite tongue-in-cheek and self-deprecating. I always do it with a little bit of comedy, while still getting across the message. 'Don't let anybody tell you that you can't still be out there, and still be sexy, and still be relevant at sixty-two.'

Back when I turned sixty, I put a post on Twitter saying, 'I'm only sixty.'

I got a flurry of responses from people saying, 'You have no idea how much I needed that today, when I was feeling old and past it . . .'

All they needed to see was somebody reversing the thinking. I learnt a lot from the Cognitive Behavioural Therapy (CBT) I had with LighterLife, when I was getting my weight under control. I used CBT techniques to give up smoking as well. Once they're in your psyche, you can use them any time.

You can either think, 'Oh, my God, I'm sixty-two today. I'm only eight years off seventy!' or you can think, 'Wow, I'm only sixty-two. Look at my dad. He's eighty-three and he's in fantastic shape.'

It doesn't work every day. We're not superhuman. We're all going to have our bad days when we feel down on ourselves, or low because something shitty has happened. But I try as much as possible to think positively, for my own well-being.

It can only be achieved with a clear mind. Again, I don't want to be the drink police and stop people having a drink on a Friday, lifting their top up and having a good time, as I used to. I'm not talking about getting tiddly and enjoying a bottle of champagne with your girlfriends. There is no doubt that being a bit merry can enhance a night. Of course it can when you're enjoying alcohol moderately and properly. But I'm just seeing more and more that it's not used like that. I have friends who don't think anything of drinking four glasses of wine a night. That's a bottle! So many people I know wake up every day feeling a little bit shit.

There's not one person I know who does dry January and doesn't say how amazing they feel, but they always go back to drinking, because they think they can't have a good time without it. And maybe they can't. Still, I look around and see people I know having really good relationships with their partners 50 per cent of the time. The other 50 per cent is spent rowing, screaming and being vile to each other, and that is purely because of alcohol.

Everybody hates a reformed drinker or a reformed smoker who rams it down your throat. I absolutely don't do that. My friends wouldn't still be my friends if I did. They love me more than ever, and I don't have any effect on their socialising. If they want to get drunk and fill their boots, then absolutely they do it. They know how important sobriety is in my life and still love a night with me when they choose to have one.

I don't say, 'Don't drink,' but they sometimes use a night out with me as an opportunity not to drink. When they get home, they will text me to say, 'What a brilliant night we had. I remember everything. I'm back home in my jammies, with a crumpet and a cup of tea, in front of the telly, and I'm going to wake up as fresh as paint tomorrow morning.'

Lincoln and I only go to a party if it is important to us. We will go early doors, stay a couple of hours and leave. Usually nobody remembers much of the party beyond the moment we leave. The next day when we ask, 'What was the rest of the night like?' people often say, 'I can't really remember, but I tell you what, I'm never drinking again.'

I completely understand, because my memories in the days when I went out and I drank were always of how bad I felt the next day, never of how great the night had been. I wish I had been more aware that I was wasting those fabulous times.

Alcohol is the only drug you have to apologise for not taking, and yet it is a very, very dangerous drug that is ruining a lot of people's potential. There are thousands of alcohol-related deaths every year, and the mortality rates are highest among the 55–69 age bracket. However, in a drinking culture, it's quite hard to contemplate sobriety. You look around and everywhere alcohol is being pushed. Where do you start when people are constantly saying things like, 'It's wine o'clock', 'It's cocktail hour somewhere in the world', 'A cheeky little wine' and 'A meal without wine is breakfast'?

Alcohol shouldn't be constantly promoted as something wonderful that adds so much joy to your life when, particularly in relationships, it can so easily just bring arguments. That's why Lincoln and I gave it up. I'm not saying we don't argue, and I'm not saying we don't say mean things to each other – we are a couple, after all! But we know how to stop it and resolve it; we're not waking up seeing a smashed plate, with no recollection of what we said to each other. If we have an argument now, we know what it's about. We remember everything that we say. It's a very different way of living your life.

These days, it boosts my self-esteem to see the look in people's eyes when I'm talking to them and engaging with them at social functions. I'm always grateful for it. The other night I was invited to a private dinner by my friend, LGBTQ activist and entrepreneur Linda Riley (we call her 'Head Lesbian of the World'), to help campaign on behalf of a female politician.

There were about fourteen of us around the table. When I arrived, Linda said, 'Would you do a little introductory speech?'

I instantly panicked. 'What the heck am I going to say?' I thought.

After Linda gave me a few pointers, I got up and said a little bit about the campaign. Then we all sat down to this wonderful, grown-up dinner.

Somebody said to me, 'I didn't realise you were so politically aware.'

'I'm not really!' I said.

What I found interesting that night was talking to people on a grassroots level. At the end of the dinner, I thought, 'If only people talked politics as we did this evening, in terms of how something will affect us and our families, as people, instead of all the jargon that you hear shouted in the House of Commons.'

I sat back in that moment and I thought, 'I'm so grateful to be here, sober and engaged. This dinner would have been a totally different experience for me, eight years ago.' I felt really grown up and quite proud of myself. These days, I feel proud of myself a lot of the time, when for a long time I really didn't.

It felt fantastic to be included in such a very grown-up evening, and to be entrusted with the introductory speech. I think this is why it's easy for me to feel that I'm 'only sixty-two,' because, since I gave up alcohol, this is the life I should have been living twenty or thirty years ago.

I would recommend sobriety to anybody who really feels that they drink too much. I'm not a believer in just cutting down. To me, evidence shows that it doesn't work if you have what you perceive as a problem with alcohol.

People say, 'I don't drink in the week.' So what? I didn't drink every day. I didn't drink every night. I never drank in the day.

'But I only drink at weekends,' they say.

Yes, but at weekends you become powerless over alcohol. You can't remember putting your kids to bed, and you can't remember the massive row that resulted in you not speaking to your husband for three days. It doesn't matter that you're not drinking Monday to Friday. Take it out of your life completely if you can. If you're reading this as a younger person and you have a problem with drink, don't wait until you're in your fifties. Try to find an anchor earlier than I did. And not everybody has to go to AA. It's great for some people, but there are other ways as well.

Being in social situations doesn't make me want to drink. For me, the only downside of being around people drinking is drunk people. You can't not be around alcohol. It's in every shop. And I always have two bottles of wine in my fridge, because I want to be able to offer my friends a drink if they want one. Do I ever think of opening them? I don't even notice that they're there. That's how little I think of alcohol. In any case, if I ever was going to drink again, not having alcohol in my house wouldn't make a difference. I've got an off-licence over the road.

The only time I think about my sobriety now is, for instance, as I'm writing this, or on a night like the night of the politician's dinner, when I thought, 'Isn't this wonderful?'

Some people need to surround themselves with a new set of sober friends when they give up drinking. Lincoln and I didn't do that, because we had each other. I had a massive advantage in having a partner to give up with me. I wish I had found an anchor earlier, but I didn't. I can't constantly look back and think, 'I wish, I wish, I wish.'

In 2020, we have different stressors from those that affected our parents' generation, and I see alcohol gradually becoming something that is used to dull the pain so people can get by. More and more, I hear people say, 'God, I've got to have a glass of wine. I need a glass of wine,' rather than, 'I can't wait to get home, pour myself a glass of wine and have some fun.'

It's time to rethink it all, and my motto is, 'It's never too late.'

A sober life is a wonderful life.

V

While writing this book, I've looked back over thirty-one years of living with a crippling, debilitating, potentially terminal illness that is still massively misunderstood by a lot of people. If you have depression, not only do you have this terrible, isolating, vile disease of the brain, but you also have to convince people you have it. Yet despite all of this and the fact that I still have it, I look back on my life to date as being a good one that I wouldn't swap. If my problems were in a pile on the floor next to twenty other people's piles, I would still choose my pile.

To those people who share my illness, I would say to them, 'Don't be defined by it. It's part of you.'

It doesn't mean you have to be grateful for it, because I'm certainly not, but I'm grateful for being given a voice to help others. Those who have it – even if they're not in the public eye like me – can still reach out, and help others, and educate them about this illness.

Over the years, I have tried to have as great an influence as possible in educating people about depression, because there are still so many people who won't talk about mental illness, and it upsets me. I have taken it on myself to be the person who takes the flak from the areas of the media that don't understand what clinical depression is, and from people who don't understand. When I received a payment for damages relating to the newspaper hacking that made my life so difficult for a decade, I spent it on making a short film about depression, *Black-eyed Susan*. It just seemed the right thing to do. More than ever, it's important to become a voice for those people who don't have one; I've done it for thirty years and will continue to do it until the day I pop my clogs.

This is an illness that happened to me because of the chemical and hormonal chaos that happened when I had a baby. I had no control over it. Everything in my garden was just fine. I still feel desperately sad for new mums with post-natal depression. In those early days, you're living in a weird world anyway. You look at your children and think, 'Where did they come from? How are they here? Are they mine?'

Everything is so different and exhausting, and coupled with this disease, this illness that makes everything seem even weirder, it is hardcore being a new mum.

When I have episodes now, I go into them with the same set of circumstances as when I come out of them. There's nowt I can do. I live with depression but I won't be defined by it. Since no mental health expert has all the answers – it falls to me and my fellow sufferers to help people understand this illness. We are a tribe and we are in this together. We need to keep talking about it and not be embarrassed about it in order to make change.

I sometimes give talks about mental illness and how employers can help their staff in the workplace. I did a speech in 2016 at Roche pharmaceutical company, and disregarding the fact that it's a big drugs company, I was impressed by their approach to workplace wellness. At their head office in Welwyn Garden City, they were having a physical wellness week, followed by a mental wellness week. They asked me to go and be their key speaker. I get a bit nervy about doing speeches as 'me', but I said I would, because I was impressed with how they had got behind their workforce and were offering such a good example to other companies.

After I did my speech, I was taken into an office where people could come and speak to me one-to-one. I felt like Dr Den! As I looked at the snaking queue of people who all wanted to talk to me, from the cleaners to top oncologists, I kept saying, 'I'm not medically qualified, you know!'

Lincoln stood on my left. 'What's going on?' he said, incredulous.

'I've got no idea,' I said, and then 'Hello,' as the next one came in.

It was amazing! I spoke to a top oncologist who was in charge of clinical trials in Europe. He'd had to decide which people in the whole of Europe could have a new breast cancer trial, and it was a huge pressure on him. I spoke to people who'd had post-natal depression and wanted to know more about hormonal treatment; I reassured people with depression who were scared about taking antidepressants.

Not only was it fantastic that that company had paid for me to give a speech, but they had also given everybody in the whole business the Headspace app, a calming mindfulness app that can help if you're feeling anxious. They had a couple of wonderful meditation spaces downstairs, where people could take half an hour out of their working day if they felt overwhelmed. They could just go downstairs and put their Headspace app on, without having to get permission or give a reason. The company also had massage therapists in once a week to help people relax. They were doing quite a lot to look after the mental well-being of their staff.

It would be lovely to see more of that in workspaces throughout the country, because knowing that your employers care is half the battle. It makes it so much less frightening to tell them that you're suffering from mental illness.

Fear can really hold people back, but don't be afraid to go to your doctor for help. Don't be afraid to talk about what you're going through. If no one in your family is listening to you, then go to a group. There are so many organisations out there, and we are so lucky now to have a way to find them. I never had any of that. In the beginning, I had no books, or people talking about it on television. I had to navigate this world completely on my own. There were no doctors who could tell me whether I'd have this illness for ever, what really it was or what its origins were. These were all things that I discovered myself.

Now we live in an age where we have access to information and help at the touch of a fingertip. If you Google 'depression groups in my area', 'depressives anonymous' or even 'what is post-natal depression?' there are answers. You will always find somewhere there are people who understand what you're going through.

Be kind to yourself. When I first started to have significant numbers of days when I felt okay again, and maybe I'd get a three-month window of wellness, I was so thrilled that I felt well that I started taking on too much. I remember my family saying, 'You'll get overwhelmed!'

I'm still doing it, although I try to be kinder to myself. 'Just give yourself another couple of days,' I think.

Yet, despite all of the positive steps I have taken – giving up drinking, not taking drugs, having hormone replacement therapy, learning CBT and mindfulness – and the fact that they have massively helped my illness, I still get episodes. Taking positive steps can reduce your episodes or lighten them, but I can't say they're a cure-all, and that's why this book is about surviving this illness, not about curing it.

A good day now is, to me, a normal day. It's not about striving to be happy – and that's why I'm against calling anti-depressants 'happy pills' and reading books with titles like *How to be Happy*. It's normalcy that I crave, and the ability to feel sad or feel happy according to my circumstances. The highs are great but I mainly like having the ability to wake up and feel normal – that's my happiness. Just feeling normal is a joy.

I hope this might be a book that people keep forever. If your friends and family don't understand your illness, give them a copy too, I want it to be a book that, even if it's just a chapter or a paragraph that they relate to, they can turn to it in times of need and remember that they will always come through it, that the visitor will always leave.

A few words from my family and friends

I asked my family and friends what it was like to have someone close who suffered from depression. Here's what they said . . .

Vin (Dad)

I will never forget the weekend when Denise's mum, Annie, and I went down to see the new baby. It was our first grandchild and we were so thrilled and excited. It had been a long and difficult delivery, but when we arrived, there was little Matthew, right as rain, and Denise was fine and Tim was over the moon, of course.

Tim and I went off to play golf, leaving a happy mother, baby and nanna. When we came back, the world had changed and Denise was in bed, feeling absolutely terrible, with no milk to give the baby. It was such a shock that we couldn't really take it in. It wasn't something we were prepared for or knew how to help, and the rest of the weekend was very traumatic.

After a couple of days, I had to go back up to the north-east to go to work, but Annie stayed down in London with Denise. Annie took Denise to see her GP, who said, 'I had five children, dear, I just didn't have time to get depressed.'

We couldn't believe it. Tim was away working and we didn't want to leave Denise in London. 'You can't stay here, pet,' we said, and brought her home to the north-east.

Depression was hardly spoken about thirty years ago, but Annie knew what Denise was going through because she was a mental health nurse and had experienced mild post-natal depression after having Denise. That made a huge difference, and we also had a sympathetic, supportive GP locally, but it was still very hard for Denise. She looked gaunt in those early days, when Matthew was first born.

The illness was with Denise severely for quite a while, off and on, until it gradually started to diminish. In time she learned how to cope with it coming and going, but we couldn't help worrying that the pain might one day be too much for her to bear. It was always in the back of my mind when she was poorly. 'I hope she never loses the plot,' I'd think. 'I hope nothing happens to her.'

Thankfully, it never did.

I have nothing but the most unbelievable admiration for the way Denise has handled having depression for all these years. I remember her calling us from Edinburgh in the early 1990s, when she was doing the play, *And A Nightingale Sang*. She was in an absolutely terrible state. 'I don't think I can go on tonight, Dad,' she said.

'You'll have to cancel, then, pet,' I said.

'But I feel so guilty!' she said.

I tried to reassure her. 'You can't help being poorly. Just try to get some rest. Anyway, we all love you and hope you'll feel better tomorrow.'

Later, Denise's friend Ian rang. 'We knew how poorly she was but she wouldn't let us cancel the show,' he said. 'She went on stage and somehow got through it.'

Denise managed to carry on for the rest of the week, which shows her amazing strength. What she has achieved in her lifetime as a successful actress is incredible. For a normal person to achieve what she has achieved, without any health problems, would deserve praise, but to achieve it with the pressure of her illness is something else. Sometimes it comes on while she's onstage, but she still manages to act as if she's laughing and joking like a normal person. It's fantastic, really. I can't praise her enough.

In later years, she didn't always let us know when she was having an episode, but Annie could tell, just by seeing her on television. We'd be watching Denise on *Loose Women*, chatting away on the panel as if she didn't have a care in the world, and Annie would say, 'She's going through it again.'

I couldn't see it the way Annie could, so I'd ring Denise after the show. 'Your mum said you weren't looking so good on *Loose Women*. Are you feeling all right, pet?'

'Not really,' she'd say. 'I've got it again.'

I always felt so bad for her. It's such an awful illness.

Denise's drinking caused a rift with her sister, Debbie, who couldn't cope with the way Denise behaved when she was a wild thing in London. I never thought the drinking was as serious as Debbie did and she got very frustrated when I defended Denise. The sisters had their problems, but they're very close and have always been supportive of one another. People often comment on how close our family is and how blessed we are in that way.

The big turning point in Denise's illness came when she went to see the Harley Street doctor, Professor Studd, and he said that the problem was her oestrogen levels, rather than her progesterone. It was a shock to think that she might have been suffering needlessly over the years. After Professor Studd began treating her, she never got the depression as badly again – and it appears to come even less frequently since she met Lincoln and gave up drinking. I'm glad to say that she seems happier now than she's ever been.

A poem I wrote for Denise . . .

I love you as you are
Not because you're a star
Cos you're my little girl
And to me you are a pearl

I love you when you're funny
And when you are sunny
I love you when you are a clown
But also when you are down

I know you have a big life
And often there is some strife
But through it all your will to win
Helps you take it on the chin

I know your sister has her fears
That drink and drugs will end in tears
But she can't understand the mind
That takes you when you must unwind

She knows how much she owes to you
And just wants to help you to come through
We love you so much with all our heart
And I promise you we'll all play our part

Dad x

Louis (son)

As a young kid, it was kind of hard to understand what was
going on when my mum got ill. She didn't have a cold and

wasn't being sick, which are the signs a seven-year-old would typically look for. Yet although I didn't have much of an understanding of the illness of depression, I was very aware that, whatever it was, it had a huge effect on my mum, and we would never know how long it would last.

By the age of about seven or eight, I knew how to act when Mum was depressed. I made sure I was very careful about what I said. Mum has always been a sensitive mum, in the sense that she loves us dearly, but she was especially sensitive about anything to do with me or my brother when she was in her drinking days and depressed.

Mum's depression will never go away, and that's something she has to deal with. I had difficulty understanding the literal effect that it had on her, but as I started to get older I noticed that it was something she couldn't control. It shocked me that it could be brought on by absolutely nothing. Mum would be fine when I went off to school, but then I'd come home and she'd be in bed in the dark, completely out of it.

It was hard to deal with, but it became a lot easier when Mum stopped drinking and found Lincoln. I believe that Lincoln is the driving force behind her recovery and sobriety. He really changed her life and in doing so, he changed ours. My brother and I both say that it makes us feel a lot better knowing that Lincoln is at home with Mum when she's going through her rough patches. I don't think my brother used to have that feeling of assurance when Mum was still with my dad, or still drinking. Matthew had a different experience from me with regard to Mum's drinking days, because he was in his late teens when it was probably at its worst, so he was dealing with it as an adult, where I was observing it as someone who didn't really understand what was going on.

Matthew and I haven't spoken about it much, but we often say how happy we are that Lincoln has come into our lives. I wouldn't say Mum's a new person now – she takes quite a lot of pride in the fact that her dearest friends all think that she's completely the same Denise – but she's just a happier, healthier, more loving friend than maybe she was ten years ago. As much as Lincoln probably wouldn't want to take all the credit for that, I really believe that he has completely changed our family's lives for the better.

Matthew (son)

One of the things you learn if somebody close to you has depression that comes on endogenously is not to take it personally. It's difficult, because your sense of self is fundamentally instilled in you from your interpersonal relationships with the people closest to you, so when it feels like there's a disconnect it can be hard to deal with it. As a young person looking up, it's sometimes difficult to be strong for your parents, but my experience of Mum's depression didn't install any trauma in me. I learned a lot of empathy, which has made it an important life lesson for me.

I think we're very lucky, because we have a liberal, understanding family unit and there's no shame around mental illness among us. It's where my parents come from culturally: there was never any shame around sexuality or self-expression, and Mum's depression was never seen as being awkward or an elephant in the room. It was something we could deal with because we had an open dialogue as a family.

Patience is a virtue when it comes to dealing with people with mental health issues because they're not experiencing time at the same rate as you are. There's often a desire to get frustrated or maybe think somebody is indulging in what they're doing, but my mum's mental health taught me and Louis that there is no time frame to happiness. The important thing is just to be there for them. You can't fix them and you can't save them, but you can maintain them when they're in that situation.

My mum sober is completely different to how she used to be. Now she's the same person consistently, instead of living with the demon that came out when she was depressed. The drink and drugs were big triggers in the cycle of her depressive episodes. In Lincoln, I know there's somebody I trust that really cares about my mum. That's all I ever wanted, and Lincoln has become a great friend of mine.

It's not necessarily anything to do with my history with my family, but I'm somebody who has also dealt with substance abuse issues and I know how incredibly hard it is to get clean, and even more so to get clean on your own terms. So I'm very proud of my mum. Most people who give up drinking without concrete support, like AA, don't stay sober, and even less so if they're giving up with a spouse who has been drinking as well. So the fact that my mum and Lincoln managed to give up alcohol and are now (at time of writing) eight years happily sober, without a desire to go back, seems incredible. It's a testament to their strong desire to prioritise relationships and structure over unhealthy, self-medicating habits.

Angie (friend)

If I had one wish in the world it would be to magic Denise's depression away. Nobody deserves to suffer with such an awful illness, least of all someone who is as special and full of life as Denise is. I've seen her in those really dark moments and it brings me to tears to think about it, because I love her so much. She's such a brilliant, kind, generous and thoughtful soul. She'll do anything for anyone, which just seems to make it more unfair.

Denise has been very vocal about her illness, which has helped her friends know what to do when she is having an

episode of depression. Unfortunately, you can't magic someone better. All you can do, as a friend, is be there and give love
unconditionally.

So I know not to ask, 'Are you okay?' every two minutes.

I have to give Denise space and time to be on her own, knowing that it will pass, as it always does. She knows to ask for help
if she's not all right; she knows that if she needs me, I'll be there
in a heartbeat, and when she's through it, I'll still be there.
Friends need to be supportive without trying to fix things.

There's been a huge difference in Denise since she gave up
drinking. She was self-medicating, not just her depression,
but also her unhappiness with many areas of her life. I felt I
lost her a bit in those self-medicating years. There were a lot
of people around her and some of them were hangers-on,
who weren't necessarily good for her because they didn't have
her interests at heart. They thought, 'Yes, she's the life and
soul of the party!', whereas if you care about someone, you
say, 'Maybe it's time to go home now.'

Denise's sobriety has really helped with her mental health.
You don't get depression just because you're drinking, but it
definitely doesn't help, because alcohol is a depressant in
itself. I understand that you get caught up in a vicious circle
of not wanting to face anything and blotting it out, but the
hangovers and the coke comedowns just fuel the fire.

As well as Denise's sobriety, the love she and Lincoln have
for each other is very positive. After spending time with
Denise and Lincoln, I'm always buzzing about life and thinking that anything's possible. They have an amazing energy
and a great sense of humour, and they've been lucky since
they've got together, especially Lincoln with his art work and
the way it's taken off. They support each other and I imagine
they keep each other sober in a lot of ways. They're a team.

Denise is not just my friend, she's family, and it is heartbreaking to see somebody you love dearly go through an

episode of depression. What amazes me about her is not only how she gets through it and comes out the other side, but also how she tries to help other people who live with chronic depression, as well as their family and friends. I'm proud of her for the way she deals with her own challenges and then wants to help others try to understand.

I happened to see Denise's last really bad episode, when she filmed it and posted it on Twitter. Even as one of her best friends, it was very distressing to watch. I thought it was incredibly brave of her to share it and I'm so proud of her, but I don't want her to do it again; I want her to concentrate on herself and getting better next time. But that's Denise – she wants to help other people if she can, and she's always been that way.

Debbie (sister)

I was working abroad when Denise had Matthew, and when I came home she was in the midst of severe post-natal depression. Until then, there hadn't been any hint or thought of depression or any other mental illness, so it was a shock. Depression is a horrible thing and I wouldn't wish it on anybody. My sister was a different Denise to the one I'd always known.

When you love someone, it's hard seeing them suffer. What I found even harder, as the years went on, was Denise's way of dealing with her depression, by self-medicating with drink and other substances. I understand that she was unhappy and struggling to cope, and I know it's what a lot of people with depression do, but it was frustrating knowing that it was never going to help the situation, and therefore feeling that she wasn't helping herself.

Denise is one of the funniest people I know – she has never needed a drink to be hilarious. She's the best sister you could have: she's a force of nature and has a very loving, generous nature. When she started self-medicating, I felt as if I'd lost her. Not because of her depression, but because of the alcohol and drugs that went with it.

My anxious times were when Denise was drinking, rather than when she was depressed. I struggled with not being able to do anything about it when she was at her worst with the self-medicating. It was like watching a car crash happen. A lot of it was taking place in the public eye, which made me feel very protective towards Matthew and Louis, and my parents.

People were afraid of saying anything to Denise about her drinking, because her response would often be very defensive, but I was so desperate to help her that I was prepared to put up with the comeback. I tried every option and angle in trying to approach her to get her to address what was happening. 'Let's go to AA,' I said. 'Let's see a counsellor.'

I tried everything and nothing worked, which left me with a terrible sense of helplessness. It put a strain on our relationship, at times. It might have seemed like I was getting frustrated, upset and angry, but it was only because I was desperate for her to get better, without the alcohol and drugs. Nothing I said came out of a place of anger or dislike – it all came from a place of love.

My first thought when Denise got pregnant with Louis, was not, 'Fantastic, she's going to have a baby,' but, 'Fantastic, she's going to have to stop drinking.'

When she stopped for eighteen months, when Louis was about six, I felt I'd got my sister back. 'I realise now that I was trying to self-medicate,' she admitted, 'and I know it's not the answer, because my episodes come far less frequently now and I feel so much better.'

She seemed much healthier and her friendships didn't suffer at all. No one said to her, 'You're boring,' because she was a lot less boring without drink. It's only the drunk who doesn't realise how boring they are.

I'll never forget the evening she came to my house and put a bottle of prosecco on the table. It was my daughter's birthday. 'I've just started having the odd glass again,' she said. When I voiced my concern, she defensively said, 'Oh Debbie, as soon as I think I can't control it, I'll stop.'

My blood ran cold. That night, a few friends came over and it was quite clear that she was not able to control it. I said so, the next day, but she was straight on the defensive. There were many more years of self-medicating after that. Nothing could stop her, not even when my mum tried talking to her.

Alcohol dependency affects your memory and I could probably reel off many things that Denise might deny happened because, when you're the drinker, you don't remember half the things, or you block them out. I was so worried about where it was going to end, so terrified of getting a phone call to say that something had happened to Denise, that I began to attend Al-Anon, a support group for the families and friends of alcoholics. This led me to suggest that our family organised an 'intervention', an orchestrated attempt to persuade Denise to seek help with her addiction to alcohol. Unfortunately, Dad wasn't really on board, and unless you've got everybody on board, it's not going to work.

It was frustrating, because Dad would accuse me of having a go at Denise, and I'd scream and say, 'Yes, Dad, because she needs help!'

I'm not criticising Dad. As a parent, I can understand that maybe you want to ignore aspects of your children's behaviour, but it's not helpful when things are as desperate as they were. It was years before he acknowledged that Denise was an alcoholic. Mum saw things more from my point of view.

You can help and support with the depression, as much as is possible, but once a person starts self-medicating, you become helpless. I sometimes thought I was going mad, because it's that old adage: you can't help somebody until they're ready to be helped. I've read so much literature about it and it all says the same thing. I was eventually advised by my GP to detach myself from the situation due to the impact it was having on my health, which was then also impacting on my own family.

It's not easy for me to open up like this, but I'm hoping it will help anyone reading the book from the perspective of trying to support someone with a mental illness who is self-medicating: my message to them is that they need to be mindful of their own well-being.

Denise had to choose when she wanted to stop, and thank God she did get to that point in her life, because it has had such a positive impact on us as a family – on Matthew and Louis, on my children, and on my relationship with Denise. It took a little while for Denise and me to get back to where we are now. 'Forgive and forget' is a great proverb but Denise's self-medicating impacted hugely on our lives, for many years. The depression was the root, but the self-medicating caused the damage.

I often wish Mum could see Denise now, because what Mum wanted for her was everything she is now and the life she is living. I know she'd be very proud too. I love it that Denise's episodes are less frequent. She looks amazing and has great energy levels. The family couldn't be happier for her. I just hope that she continues to be able to manage the depression as she is now. I know she can't have complete control, but it's fantastic that she is doing everything she can to help herself. The effect on the whole family, especially on Matthew and Louis, is huge.

Throughout it all, hard though it was, I never stopped loving Denise. It has taken her a long time to get to this stage, but some people never do, so we've just got to be so grateful that she's where she is now. I couldn't be prouder or happier for her.

Rose (friend)

In the early days, when Denise had Matthew and developed post-natal depression, it was easier to understand, because I was aware of post-natal depression and felt I understood it a little. When it became clinical depression, it was quite hard to understand, because it wasn't affected by any circumstantial changes. It could literally come on within moments, when nothing had changed.

When Denise first got depression, my initial reaction was that it would hopefully make things better if I did X, Y or Z. I'm an 'I can make things better' sort of person, so I think, 'I'll do this,' or 'I'll do that.' But actually what Denise needs – and she says this to me now – is just to know I'm there. Whatever she wants or needs, if I can do it, I will. Just be there. Don't do anything more than that.

At first, it was really hard feeling there was nothing I could do. She was in this place where I couldn't really reach her. Over time, I realised that by doing nothing you are helping the most. You are doing what the person who needs you wants you to do.

Denise's depression has gone on for so long that it now is part of the make-up of our relationship. It's awful when she's going through an episode. You don't want your friend to be feeling the way she is feeling and sometimes I get quite upset when I think about the terrible times she's had. On the other side of the coin, I look at Denise, who is such a fabulous person, and I think, 'She is that person, encompassing all those facets.'

Denise and I have known each other since we were teenagers and she's an amazing friend. We still laugh like drains and our friendship is incredibly fun, which is wonderful. People think, 'Oh, you get into your sixties and you become these boring old people,' but we're not like that at all. We go out and have a brilliant time. Fortunately, there are larger spaces between episodes these days. Denise is very happy and I think that it helps, perhaps.

Denise giving up alcohol has been an amazing turning point for her and I completely take my hat off to her. I know how difficult it must have been because I know how entrenched alcohol was in her life. It's made a tremendous difference to her and it's wonderful to see how happy she is now that she doesn't have that addiction. She's a very, very special friend and I couldn't imagine my life without her in it.

Lincoln (husband)

I was delighted to be asked to contribute to this book, a book that shares over thirty-one years of experience of an illness that I can only describe as evil, and is misunderstood by many people. Denise is my wife, my friend and the love of my life. She is an extremely intelligent, creative woman who has a huge heart that beats to the tune of being welcoming and warm to people. She has astounded me over the years.

We met ten years ago in what we call 'the madness' and quickly formed a solid bond. Since we opened a new chapter of life together, we have become inseparable. Very early on, way before we got married, Denise explained to me about her mental illness. I found it hard to comprehend how this 'feeling low', as I saw it back then, had such a hold, both mentally and physically, over her.

I came to learn how the all-consuming nature of this disabling illness took over her entire life in all areas, crippling her. I would see it first in her eyes, as her dear mum Annie could see it, even if she was on the television. As time went by and episodes came and went, I began to understand that the illness could take my wife away from me temporarily; I also learned that the person behind the illness needs love and support and to be left to deal with it in their own way.

I would have to admit I have had times when I thought, 'I don't want this to happen right now, what about MY feelings?' But I have seldom shared these thoughts and the only way I can help Denise is to stand by her and be there if she needs me.

This book needed to be written; this woman's story of mental illness needed to be heard. I hope it will be seen as an honest, clear and accessible insight into a terrible illness, and be read not only by sufferers but also by their friends and loved ones.

Steven (friend)

When I first met Denise in the front room of a friend's house in Brighton, it was love at first sight. She was witty, gorgeous and just someone I really connected with. We also shared the same wicked sense of humour.

Our journey together has had plenty of highs and lows. It has seen us flying in private jets and dashing along exotic beaches in India (we won't touch on the low moments). Being with Denise is like being with family. Her own family treat me like one of theirs.

But what really brings us together, and what means the most to me, is the simple times – being under a duvet watching *CBB*, crying with laughter or just hanging out in our PJs. Friendships are like marriages, but often they last longer. You need to be there for the good times and the bad times, and Denise has held my hand in all my times of need.

You can be at a showbiz party filled with colourful exciting people and there she is, my friend of thirty-six years, Denise Welch, lighting up the room and making everyone feel important. She is always pleased to meet new people and will often tell you such a witty story that you cannot help but be proud even to know this remarkable woman, let alone call her your best friend. She has such an ability to please, and Denise often forgets to please herself.

On occasion, I can take my attention off her for a few minutes and, when I look back, there it is in her eyes, what she calls 'the visitor'. No one would know. She has become so accustomed to hiding it that you would have to know the signs.

I remember when it happened at a special birthday party for her sister, Debbie. Denise was hosting pre-theatre nibbles and drinks before going to see *Motown the Musical*. Everyone was excited, and Denise was making sure her sister and guests were having the best time. But Denise's energy was shifting – it is quite sensitive and she has no control over it. I really felt for her. There was nothing I could do, although it seems to help when I say, 'I know.'

It is painful to watch Denise when she is having an episode, especially when she goes on television or performs, and you can see her suffering and all you want to do is give her a hug. When she has stayed over at mine and alas the visitor comes too, just rubbing her shoulders or wrapping her in a warm blanket seems to make her feel safe.

Denise's need to please often comes at the expense of her own happiness and to the cost of those she loves. But recently, and since she has found love with the man who is her anchor, she has managed to stop and ask if what she is doing is making her truly happy. This is, in part, due to his guidance, as she has found someone who is her soulmate.

People often tell me how lucky I am to have Denise as a friend and say what fun it must be going to events with Denise, and how they can relate to her. Yes, I am lucky, although sometimes the events can actually be hard work. Of course, the fact that people relate and see themselves in her is what makes

Denise – along with her talents – so successful. But unless you have held her, looked into her eyes and seen the pain, the love and so many things that make her so unique and special, you will never really know how remarkable a woman she is.

Pam (friend)

I knew Denise before she was pregnant with Matthew, when we were partygoers and she was the funniest friend I knew, as she still is. It sounds dramatic, but the depression took her life; it literally sucked the life out of her and it was just awful for us to watch. I didn't really understand it at first, because I didn't get post-natal depression with either of my kids. However, about six months after Matthew was born, I lost my mum very suddenly and very tragically and suffered a clinical depression brought on by a shock, which gave me some idea of what Denise had gone through. The difference was that my depression obviously passed, with medication and seeing a psychiatrist, whereas Denise's has lasted for the rest of her life.

I could always tell when Denise was having a bad day on *Loose Women* – I could see it in her eyes. She would smile and do her job, but you could see there was no light in her eyes. And when I spoke to her on the phone, I knew it – all she had to say was 'Hello' and I'd know. It was as if somebody had let the air out of a balloon: the eyes were dead; there was no sing-song in her voice.

Depression is a horrible, vile illness, because it steals your friends away from you, if only for a little while. It's torture for all of us who have known her for over thirty years to watch her go through it. Thank God it's less frequent these days. However, she has relapses and it's awful. One of the worst times for me was when she was doing *Celebrity Big Brother*. I just wanted to get a helicopter and fly in and pluck her out of there. I cried for the full three weeks she was on there. She was sad and trying not to let it show; she was depressed and trying not to be. It was heartbreaking.

Denise is the best company and the funniest person you could ever be with. She makes me laugh every single day. We're both nutcases when it comes to reality TV and I can simply text one word – 'Shahs', referring to the TV programme *Shahs of Sunset* – and she'll come back with 'OMG, who else apart from me would know what that meant?'

It's an amazing relationship, and so special. However, it's difficult watching your friend go through lifelong depression. It's torture for her and it's torture for her friends, because there is nothing we can do about it. People say, 'Pull yourself together' and 'Buy yourself a new dress', but it's not about that – it's not about anything at all. It's waking up to find the blackness is there; it's like having blinkers on. No amount of joviality from friends can make it stop.

From a friend's point of view, feeling helpless has been the worst aspect of Denise's illness. Not being able to help your friend is awful. She doesn't reach out to us because she can't – what can she say? 'I'm having a bad day'? We already know it. We can hear it in her voice and there's nothing we can do; and she withdraws. Thankfully, she's got Lincoln there and it's fantastic that he understands it. Tim also understood it, thank God.

It's so much better now and I'm so happy for Denise that she deals with it a lot better than she used to. Obviously, she's on the right path and getting the right treatment, but for many years she wasn't and it was awful to watch her self-medicate with drink and drugs. I don't think we realised she was doing that a lot of the time. Rose and I are the friends who have known her the longest and when we look back on our 'Tres Amigo' days when we were the Three Musketeers, we didn't really see it. It's only in retrospect that we realise that she was unhappy for much of the time. She was making it all go away by drinking and being the fun party person, but obviously dying inside.

I've had other friends who have gone through depression and because I've seen what Denise has gone through, I've been able to be there and recognise it before it's taken hold. That's been brilliant. Denise has helped people in so many ways.

A Look Back At How Far We've Come

One of the reasons I wrote *The Unwelcome Visitor* was to reassure people who were struggling with depression that they weren't alone. I was hoping to reach those who hadn't necessarily come by the help they've needed, perhaps because they'd found it hard to access mental health services, or because they didn't feel strong enough to accept help or know how to talk about how they were feeling. It makes a world of difference to realise that someone else understands what you're going through and I wanted to encourage people to keep going and believe in getting better, as my mum always encouraged me when I first became poorly.

But who could have guessed, in September 2019, when I shared a video of myself in the middle of a depressive episode, that the book I would go on to write about my illness would be published at the height of a global pandemic? Who knew that we would be in the midst of an incredibly stressful, at times traumatic, upsetting and overwhelming year that would create mental health issues for many more people than normal life does? Never in a million years did I imagine that anything as momentous and horrible could happen.

Mental health services suddenly became harder than ever to access, leaving many people feeling anxious, isolated and needing help – and the timing of *The Unwelcome Visitor* started to seem very fortuitous, aimed as it was at anyone who might be finding it hard to cope or was feeling unsupported. I've been moved and humbled by the reaction to the book. People have written to me to say that it has saved their life, or their mum's or their sister's life, which is a very, very dramatic thing to say but I understood exactly what they meant because having your illness recognised is sometimes what it takes. I've received messages from all over the world, including countries where the book hasn't been published but people were gifted it and have shared it, which is great to hear, as I always wanted it to be a book that was shared and passed on.

'I've been poorly for 25 years and never in all that time had my illness explained in the way you've explained it,' people have told me.

One of the chapters most commented on was the one with contributions from my friends and family. People appreciated the way it shone a light on the under-represented group of people who live with and love those with depression. Soon after the book was published, I became an ambassador for the mental health charity, Sane, and got involved with a campaign called Breaking Depression, which is about highlighting major depressive disorder – or clinical depression – and trying to teach people the difference between mental health issues and mental illness. Lincoln's contribution to *The Unwelcome Visitor* led to him coming on board with the campaign to talk about how people can help their loved ones when they can't help themselves. The next thing we knew we were appearing together on programmes like the *Channel 5 News* and ITV's *Lorraine*.

Lincoln very openly says that he didn't know anything about clinical depression before he met me. He now realises how serious it is and that there's nothing of an indulgence about it. 'When Denise is depressed, I try to listen to her, clear her diary and make sure that she's alone if she wants to be alone,' he always says. 'It's important to understand that this is a severe illness.'

People became very good at using online ways of communicating during 2020 and there is a new digital world of mental health support out there. But when you are in a depression and someone says, 'Go on a website,' they might as well be saying, 'Run a marathon!'

You can't go on a website. You are in a catatonic state and can't take anything in. This is where the supporter's role can be crucial – where the Lincolns of the world come in. When you can't go online for yourself, they can find help for you at the click of a Google button or with a bit of research; anything from online support groups and like-minded communities to one-to-one therapy, or simply the latest mental health information.

Although many of us are sick of the word Zoom and can't wait to have human contact again, for people who are mentally ill or have mental health issues, it can be a life saver. A lot of people with anxiety would never go to a support group physically because they couldn't leave the house, but they will go to one on Zoom – and it might keep them afloat until they can enter the mainstream world of mental health treatment, if there is a delay.

I've seen people hook up on social media as a result of my story. Everybody was at home when *The Unwelcome Visitor* was published and that gave them more time and space to read, listen and comment online. Readers started sharing experiences – and when the restrictions were lifted in the summer they were able to meet up.

'You seem like you really understand, Susie, and I've just seen that you're just down the road in Coventry!'

Making an Instagram Live video has become a popular way of reaching out. Saying, 'My name is Joan, I suffer from depression and I'm going to be doing an Instagram Live,' is a lot easier if you're saying it into a camera in your living room than in front of a room full of people, and even if four viewers watch it, that's four people you've befriended and helped.

If you're stuck at home, there's a wealth of online resources to get people painting, drawing, cooking, gardening, writing, sewing and a hundred other things. If you're in a major depressive disorder episode, you will probably not feel up to doing anything, but when you are out of it and perhaps having periods of feeling overwhelmed but not in that catatonic state, a supporter can help you find something that you'd like to try. Creativity reduces anxiety and stress in a very natural way, and has been shown to help people process trauma. Even just a bit of knitting can release dopamine, your natural anti-depressant.

Anxiety was not new to me, or to a lot of people who'd had mental health issues before the advent of Covid 19, and so some of us felt we were in a better position than others to cope with the stress and worry of the pandemic. For years I'd woken up with that stomach-churning feeling you associate with traumatic times, despite having no reason to feel that way, and so I already had at my fingertips some of the tools that would lessen its impact. I've had to do a lot of self care and practise what I preach with regard to looking after myself, and strategies like deep breathing, meditation and exercise all helped me to stay balanced and be a support to my family and friends.

Have there been moments when I've felt overwhelmed? Yes. Have I woken up and spent the day crying? Yes, many times! But several of my mates had a worse time of it than I did, including friends who had always been supportive of me and my illness, despite never understanding it.

As they panicked about their health, jobs, futures and the safety of their loved ones, some of them experienced levels of anxiety that they had never imagined possible.

'What's the difference between your illness and how I'm feeling now?' one of my colleagues asked me. 'Because I have never in my life felt so frightened that I don't feel in control of my mental health.'

Anxiety can reach such an extreme point that it tips over and becomes clinical depression – and then it can be there for life. We saw a lot of this in 2020, with people who would never have had a mental illness becoming extremely mentally unwell because they weren't able to draw on the resources, or access the treatment, that those who have suffered before know of.

Just like everybody else, I've felt emotional and traumatised at times, but only as a normal person reacting to a surreal and unexpected set of circumstances, I'm relieved to say – not as somebody in the thick of a major depressive disorder.

I haven't had another episode since the one that spawned this book, which just shows that clinical depression is not necessarily tied to circumstances. A year and a half is a long time for someone like me to feel normal; if my depression was reactive rather than endogenous, then I would certainly have become ill.

There was a point towards the end of 2020 when it kept coming into my mind, just because I was very aware of how long it had been. 'Oh no, I'm going to bring it on by thinking about it too much!' I thought, as usual.

But the unwelcome visitor didn't come.

Things would have been very different if he had, because my illness is ruinous and horrendous when he enters the house and I often can't do much to help myself, let alone others. Still, as I constantly say, he will always leave, and in between episodes, my life can be great. I don't mean great as in joyous and doing high kicks up the road – at least, not during the terrible times we've been having. I mean being well enough to grasp life with both hands, which is something I've been trying my hardest to do. I wrote *The Unwelcome Visitor* partly to show that you don't need to be defined by depression or allow it to stop you living your life between episodes. You can move forward from it, just as we can all move forward from the pandemic, sooner or later.

Working on the book took me back to a dark past that I hadn't wanted to revisit, but it also showed me how much mental strength I've gained from learning how to live with major depressive disorder, which has helped me flip the narrative of age.

To any of my older readers who are feeling down on themselves and think they're on the scrapheap, I'd like to say, 'You're not!'

I'm proof of the pudding: I'm still here. I'm still relevant. I'm still being quoted and doing my job. Age is often just a point of view – and I've reached a point where I've realised that I can either think, 'Oh my God, I'm 62, I'm going to be 70 in eight years,' or I can think, 'I'm only 62. I might have a good 20 or 30 years ahead of me.'

I'm busier than ever, which is quite something for someone who has suffered from debilitating clinical depression for 31 years. Yes, my illness comes and floors me, but even when it does, nothing is going to stop me once the unwelcome visitor leaves.

The first lockdown was very busy at the beginning for us actors, because so many charities were calling on us to help present information online, which I was very glad to do. And since I wasn't able to go out on a book tour when *The Unwelcome Visitor* was released, most of the publicity I did for the book took place at home. I was constantly on the television in the kitchen! Lincoln would walk in of a morning, wearing hardly anything at all, and do a double-take as he found me sat chatting in front of a ring light, with the clothes maiden winched out of sight of the camera and piles of washing up shoved to one side of the sink. If it wasn't one thing, it was another: publicising the book, highlighting a good cause or appearing on *Loose Women*.

It actually feels important to the morale of the country to keep programmes like *Loose Women* and the soap operas on the television, because people need some normality and consistency, and it's amazing how these shows have adapted to this Covid world, for now. A few of the *Loose Women* panellists don't like doing the programme from home – and it's definitely not as good, because you don't feel as much a part of it – but I'll take it because at least I'm still managing to do it. As you'd expect, we've been talking a lot about Covid 19 on the panel, but also about important issues like Black Lives Matter, which has really helped to make a difference and raise awareness. The time to confront the troubles of our black friends at home and around the world is long overdue.

I've been very grateful for the work that's come my way. A few weeks into the first lockdown of 2020, Julie Graham, a friend of mine and an amazing actress, rang me up and said, 'I've been working on this idea for a couple of years and we were just about to start pitching it to networks, but that's not happening right now. I just wondered – I've got this great part of Doll and I thought maybe we could try and do something in lockdown?'

She sent me the script and I was hooked - and so were the rest of the brilliant cast that assembled: Tracy Ann Oberman, Tamzin Outhwaite, Angela Griffin, Alison Newman and Nimmy March. Exploring the lives and relationships of a group of women, *Dun Breedin'* was a ten-part drama made up of ten-minute episodes that took a completely new look at the menopause. Doll, my part, was the mother in law from hell.

Nobody could meet up, so we rehearsed on Zoom with our wonderful female director, Robin Shepperd, and filmed each episode at home. Lincoln was my director of photography and when the producers spotted an acting spark in him he became my co-star and played my on-screen partner. Who knew? It was fantastic to do it and we were all really proud of how it turned out.

Acting jobs are like buses and before I knew it I was offered the opportunity to create the fabulous character of Trish in the long-running Channel 4 soap opera, *Hollyoaks*. 'We so hope Denise is going to say yes to this,' the producers told my agent, 'because as soon as we started creating the character, we felt it had Denise written all over it.'

It's an actor's dream to hear those words and now I'm playing Trish I can see what they mean. Trish is my age and has a lover who's 45, and yet that's not the main issue, which is fabulous. Her first line when she walks in is, 'No one ignores a booty call from me.'

What a brilliant line for a woman in her sixties – I'm so proud of *Hollyoaks* for coming up with it.

Trish's boyfriend, Brad, is a real player and there's no way he's faithful to her. That's fine with me, but I needed to be clear with the producers that he's not with her for any other reason than that he fancies her. And they said, 'Absolutely!'

Sadly, we can't show the attraction physically because we're filming within Covid guidelines, but it's there in the writing and quite clear in the looks they exchange that they have a very active sex life. I love that, because women in their sixties are never written about as if they're still active sexually. At the time of writing, I've been filming for six weeks but at no point do we mention how old Trish is. She's clearly older than him and that's it.

It's great to think of people watching *Hollyoaks* and thinking, 'Look at Trish! She's got a bloody younger man. Look at her go in with her booty call.'

I never thought I'd be doing a soap again – I didn't think I'd have the stamina to do it – but actually I'm fine with getting up at five in the morning to go to work in the dark; I love the role so much that I'm getting up with a spring in my step.

I've also been filming a show that's currently called *Surviving Evil with Denise Welch*. It's on the Crime and Investigation channel, which is my favourite channel; anyone who knows me knows that I'm obsessed with real life crime. I got together with a production company and we pitched the idea for the show at the beginning of lockdown. It's about people who have experienced the trauma of a real life crime and don't consider themselves to be victims, but survivors. It's been absolutely fascinating meeting them and hearing their inspiring stories.

So at the time of writing this, I'm juggling three jobs and feeling incredibly lucky, but also being very careful not to take on too much. Much as I count my blessings, especially when it comes to my family, I've found it really hard to bear what's happened to the world in the past year. I have a tendency to be too much of an empath, which makes life difficult, so I have to make sure I look after myself mentally and physically and I would encourage readers to do the same.

I've had to learn from Lincoln, who only needs to take one look at me to see when I'm becoming overwhelmed by the state of the world. 'Pull back, put your phone down,' he says. 'You can't do anything about this right now.'

He's had to be quite strict with me, because I was at one point getting myself far too involved, watching awful things about how lonely and isolated old people were becoming in care homes and worrying about young people, carers and key workers.

'You're going to go down,' Lincoln warned me.

We stopped watching the news. Even though I am a panellist on a topical news programme and have an obligation to know what's going on, I also have to know my limits. Often the mainstream news just upsets me too much.

It's good to have a sense of what's good and bad for your personal mental health, and I've realised that helping other people is good for mine, even if it's just getting some shopping for somebody. Any little thing helps. Last week, I judged the Gingerbread House competition at Kingsclear Care Home in Surrey; this Friday I'm going to be in the Zoom audience at their care home awards. Ever since I got into a conversation with Helen Rooke, the care home's Deputy Manager, on Twitter, I've tried to make sure that I check in with the residents every Friday, as much for my own sanity and mental wellbeing as for theirs. It's very much a two-way thing, as I've just felt so traumatised by the idea of old people not being able to see their families through the pandemic, and the antidote, for me, is seeing a home where they're doing everything in their power to fill the gap left by loved ones and make the residents feel loved and looked after. I'd really recommend connecting with a care home, as it has done me a lot of good. You don't have to be famous – anybody can write to their local care home to ask, 'Is there somebody that doesn't have anybody? Because maybe I could talk to them once a week?'

I'm fortunate to have Lincoln as a supporter, because I don't always follow my own advice when it comes to keeping a balance. There's obviously a dark side to social media and I tell people to stay off it sometimes and to stay away from the clickbait media, but I myself have days when I don't. I always regret it, like yesterday, when I clicked on an article online. Some papers seem to relish the doom and gloom of the pandemic and you can lose all hope and the will to live within the first few paragraphs you read. I shouldn't have done it, but I did, and then spent yesterday in tears at the thought of how things are going to get worse before they get better.

It's about knowing what's best for you. Despite the downsides of social media, it can be a huge force for good if you find the right corners. People seem to be using it more to discuss mental health issues than holidays and clothes now, which is a big plus, especially for those who can't go out or don't want to go out because they're poorly. I know that a lot of young people who already had anxiety started to feel calmer when the world locked down, because they weren't picking up Instagram and seeing this or that person's glamorous life, with planes and parties and designer clothes. They were free of the urge to compare and despair, at least for a time.

Not everyone was able to stay home and bake banana bread, though. As we know, the pandemic has caused desperate poverty and it's the cruellest thing that could have happened to those people living on the breadline. Yet a lot of young people said to me that they felt relieved that they couldn't be looking for a job that they were terrified to get because of their anxiety. Nobody was saying to them, 'You've got to get yourself out there. You've got to get a job and go to work!'

They were split into two camps, as I could see. Although it's been great for some people's mental health to be able to take their foot off the accelerator, it's been really heartbreaking to see the effects on others in terms of their lives, jobs and futures. It's not just the young and the elderly – it's everyone. I have a GP friend who is very concerned about the number of middle aged men who have presented at her surgery or online with suicidal thoughts. They're the very people who are least likely to ever open up about their mental health, but in the midst of the pandemic, when they've lost their job and their marriage collapses, what begins as a mental health issue can very quickly become a severe mental illness.

Hopefully, people are starting to realise that we need to treat mental health on a par with physical health. We need to invest far more in this country's mental health services. People have to speak out about it and I'm prepared to shout from the rooftops. The pandemic highlighted how inadequate our mental health services are. Surely it's time for change and I hope reading this book has encouraged you to join me on that mission!

Acknowledgements

My husband Lincoln for saving me.

My sons Matty, Louis and Lewis for making me the proudest mum in the world.

My dad Vin for showing us all that life is for living and that being 83 is no excuse for slowing down!!

Debbie, my sister. Thank you for always being there when many would have walked away.

My nieces and nephew, Olivia, Alex and Wills. I love you like my own.

My mum-in-law Jenny for filling a mum-sized hole in my heart.

Duncan, the not-so-little brother I never had!

Rose, Pammie, Steven and Ang. My best friends who have been by my side throughout the last 30 years.

Gordon Wise for believing in me.

Briony Gowlett for having faith that my story could help others.

Bex Elliff, my acting agent who always puts my wellness before my career.

And finally, Rebecca Cripps. By my side for 10 years and without whom you wouldn't be reading this book.

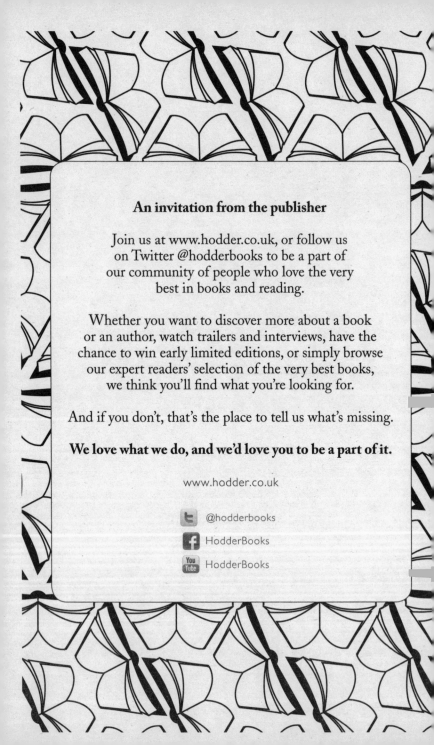

An invitation from the publisher

Join us at www.hodder.co.uk, or follow us
on Twitter @hodderbooks to be a part of
our community of people who love the very
best in books and reading.

Whether you want to discover more about a book
or an author, watch trailers and interviews, have the
chance to win early limited editions, or simply browse
our expert readers' selection of the very best books,
we think you'll find what you're looking for.

And if you don't, that's the place to tell us what's missing.

We love what we do, and we'd love you to be a part of it.

www.hodder.co.uk

@hodderbooks

HodderBooks

HodderBooks